Passport to Successful Outcomes
for Patients Admitted to ICU

Carole Boulanger · David McWilliams
Editors

Passport to Successful Outcomes for Patients Admitted to ICU

Meeting Patient Goals of Care

Second Edition

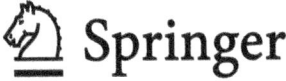 Springer

Editors
Carole Boulanger
Intensive Care Unit
Royal Devon University NHS Foundation
Exeter, Devon, UK

David McWilliams
Centre for Care Excellence
Coventry University
Coventry, UK

ISBN 978-3-031-53018-0   ISBN 978-3-031-53019-7   (eBook)
https://doi.org/10.1007/978-3-031-53019-7

This Springer imprint is published by the registered company Springer Nature Switzerland AG
The registered company address is: Gewerbestrasse 11, 6330 Cham, Switzerland

If disposing of this product, please recycle the paper.

Foreword

In the ever-evolving landscape of intensive care medicine, where each single patient's journey through critical illness is as unique as the individual themselves, the significance of comprehensive, multidisciplinary care cannot be overstated. As we navigate the complexities of ICU environments, it becomes increasingly apparent that successful patient outcomes hinge not only on technological advancements but, more crucially, on the collaborative efforts of dedicated healthcare professionals. This human chain is absolutely remarkable.

The second edition of "Passport to Successful ICU Discharge" stands as a testament to this collective commitment to excellence. Under the skilled editorship of Carole Boulanger and David McWilliams, whose unbeatable dedication to research and patient care has set a standard for excellence, this volume delves deeper into the intricacies of ICU management, offering invaluable insights and evidence-based practices for optimising patient recovery.

In the wake of the unprecedented challenges posed by the COVID-19 pandemic, the importance of effective critical care has been thrust into the spotlight. In his foreword to the first edition, Maurizio Cecconi's poignant reflection on the essence of ICU practice resonates profoundly, reminding us that beyond the ventilators and monitors lies the beating heart of intensive care—the compassionate collaboration of nurses, allied healthcare professionals, and clinicians.

"Passport to Successful Outcomes for Patients Admitted to ICU" transcends the traditional confines of medical literature, offering a holistic framework for guiding patients through every stage of their ICU journey. From the meticulous attention to detail during admission to the comprehensive rehabilitation strategies aimed at promoting independence and quality of life, each chapter encapsulates the essence of patient-centred care. The multidisciplinary approach embraced within these pages reflects a fundamental shift in our understanding of critical illness—a recognition that true healing extends beyond the physical realm to encompass the emotional, psychological, and social dimensions of recovery. As we strive to create environments conducive to healing, the significance of effective communication, infection prevention, and psychological support emerges as indispensable pillars of care.

In essence, "Passport to Successful Outcomes for Patients Admitted to ICU" serves as both a beacon of guidance and a testament to the unrestricted dedication of ICU professionals worldwide. Its pages resonate with the collective wisdom of clinicians, researchers, and caregivers, united in their pursuit of excellence and never-ending commitment to patient well-being.

As we embark on this journey through the corridors of critical care, may this volume serve as a guiding light, illuminating the path towards successful patient outcomes and reaffirming our shared commitment to compassionate, evidence-based practice.

President European Society of Intensive Care Medicine   Elie Azoulay
Chef de Service de Médecine, Intensive & Reanimation
Hopital St Louis,
Paris, France

Preface

In 1892, Dr. William Osler in wrote,

it is much more important to know what sort of a patient has a disease than what sort of a disease a patient has.

This sentiment still very much holds true today. The past few decades has seen increasing numbers of patients admitted to critical care units, with high acuity of illness and an increasingly complex array of comorbidities. Thankfully technological advancements and developments in care delivery mean survival rates have improved. However, with limited resources and stretched healthcare systems, there is a risk that critical care becomes focused on the completion of tasks, losing sight of the individuality of the person receiving that care.

A passport is well recognized as one of the earliest known documents certifying the identity and key details of the bearer, primarily for the purposes of safe passage of travel and return home at the end of a journey. Whilst no patient or their family would choose an intensive care journey, the principles of safe passage do hold true in this context and the goal is always a safe return home. The concept of a "passport" for a critically ill patient therefore comprises the key aspects of care and management to enable safe passage. Avoidance of complications and the early establishment of a relationship between the patient, their family, and the multi-professional team can have a significant impact on how the ICU journey progresses. Person-centred care is at the heart of the intensive care journey and is valued among the intensive care community—how far it reaches into busy intensive care units is less easy to quantify.

Passport to Successful Outcomes for Patients Admitted to ICU-Meeting Goals of Care has been created to highlight key aspects of intensive care from admission through to discharge. Written by an expert multi-professional team of nurses and key therapists from across the world, the ICU patient journey is presented through the lens of individual experts making up the critical care team. The intention is to signpost how focusing the spotlight on the patient as a whole can contribute to a successful return of patients to their previous lives and families or facilitate a peaceful and dignified death. The authors present the latest evidence, emphasising the attention to detail necessary to avoid ICU-related complications, coupled with ensuring that care is person-centred. This edition builds on our first text *Passport to*

Successful Discharge and provides a timely update reflecting the challenges and innovations of the last couple of years. In addition, it is also acknowledged that for some patients admitted to critical care survival is not always possible. A new chapter has now been included to consider how holistic, multidisciplinary care is for the person at the end of their life.

This is by no means an exhaustive text, but one which views the patient journey from the point of admission with the goal of ensuring a successful outcome for people admitted to critical care, whether that is returning the patient and family to their previous lives or supporting them and their family to ensure a good death. It is intended to be practical, informative, and thought provoking to ensure we maximise the expertise of the multi-professional team in the patients' interests.

Exeter, Devon, UK   Carole Boulanger
Coventry, UK   David McWilliams

Contents

The Person Before the Patient: The Importance of a Good History

1

Fiona Howroyd and Andrew Lockwood

1.1 Introduction

The Intensive Care Unit (ICU) is a complex and dynamic environment intended for the care of the critically ill patient [1]. Receiving 24-h care, patients in the ICU are carefully managed for life-threatening illness, through intricate multiorgan support and continuous monitoring [2]. In the initial stages of recovery, treatment goals may be short term, medically focused and interchangeable dependent on the patient's response. Anticipating a patient's post-acute care needs for discharge may be difficult in the ICU due to the uncertainty of recovery and the rapid changing priorities in a patient's condition [3]. However, as medical care advances, the optimisation of recovery as a therapeutic objective has developed increasing prominence rather than mere survival alone [4]. For many survivors of critical illness, their discharge from ICU is the start of an uncertain journey, facing numerous physical and non-physical problems [5]. The overall sequelae of critical illness lead to reduced quality of life amongst ICU survivors [6].

It is essential that the ICU team assesses and manages the physical and non-physical issues experienced by ICU patients as soon as possible, to optimise long-term outcomes. National guidelines in the UK serve as a useful template, recommending the completion of an early and comprehensive assessment of physical and non-physical factors which may influence recovery and long-term outcomes [4]. This assessment requires a detailed understanding of the patient's history, including their pre-admission functional and health status, helping to identify risk

F. Howroyd (✉)
University Hospitals Birmingham NHS Foundation Trust, Birmingham, UK
e-mail: fiona.howroyd@uhb.nhs.uk

A. Lockwood
Royal Devon University Healthcare NHS Foundation Trust, Exeter, Devon, UK
e-mail: andrew.lockwood@nhs.net

© The Author(s), under exclusive license to Springer Nature
Switzerland AG 2024
C. Boulanger, D. McWilliams (eds.), *Passport to Successful Outcomes for Patients Admitted to ICU*, https://doi.org/10.1007/978-3-031-53019-7_1

factors for physical and non-physical morbidity [4]. Early assessment of such potential deficits is required to inform holistic care, facilitate early rehabilitation and identify the ongoing specialist needs of survivors of critical illness, beyond their ICU discharge [4]. This chapter will therefore explore the following:

- *When* to attain a patient history in the ICU.
- *How* to attain a patient history in the ICU.
- *What* a good history should include in the ICU.
- *Why* an early, detailed history is important.

Throughout the chapter, the practicalities and challenges of taking a good history in the ICU will be considered, along with practical advice on how to overcome these challenges. The benefits of a good history will also be discussed throughout the chapter, considering how this can inform patient-centred care.

1.2   When to Attain a Patient History in the ICU

Although considered an essential component of patient-centred care, gaining a good history in the ICU can be a challenging concept for healthcare professionals [7]. Every situation is unique, yet it is important for clinicians to gauge the right time to approach patients and their relatives in a sensitive manner [8]. With the constant noise, lights and alarms of machines, the ICU environment alone is considered to be a hostile and stress-inducing place for both patients and their relatives [2]. Furthermore, there is the emotion and grief experienced as patients deal with the uncertainty of critical and life-threatening illness [9]. Gaining a detailed history about the patient in order to inform holistic rehabilitation goals may be misinterpreted at the acute stages; either giving false hope of recovery or being deemed insensitive when prognosis is uncertain [10]. A compassionate judgement is key; considering that ICU patients and their family members experience high levels of anxiety and psychological distress during the ICU admission [11, 12].

However, delays need to be avoided whilst selecting the optimal time to obtain this detailed information. As recommended by the NICE guidelines, rehabilitation needs to commence early in the ICU in order to prevent the physical and non-physical complications of critical illness. Specifically, the associated Quality Standards advise that rehabilitation goals should be set and agreed by day 4 of ICU admission [13]. At this time, patients may still be acutely unwell requiring multiorgan support. Although this may seem early, it is important to recognise patients who are critically ill for more than 4 days are at greater risk of physical and non-physical symptoms. A delay in goal setting may subsequently delay the care and rehabilitation required to overcome such negative effects. Early goal setting is therefore essential, even if preventative in nature, ensuring a well-structured holistic rehabilitation plan that is documented, communicated and executed [14].

On balance, although this would seem to be at a stressful and uncertain time for patients and their families, comprehensive assessment and detailed history taking are required in the first few days of admission, in order to inform individualised rehabilitation goals by day 4 [13]. Information gathering at such an early stage therefore requires a systematic, professional and sensitive manner [8].

1.3   How to Obtain an Effective Patient History in the ICU

As well as gauging when it is an appropriate and sensitive time to gain a good patient history, it is also important to consider the practicalities of *how*.

1.3.1   Taking a History from the Patient

The first line of approach to history taking should be from the patient themselves. This will allow the clinician to hear the patients thoughts, beliefs and priorities in their own words. Although challenging to approach in the ICU, when handled correctly, the interview process can concurrently support clinicians in developing a therapeutic relationship. Through open communication, empathy and listening skills, the clinical team is able to evoke a relationship of trust and understanding. This may be reassuring for both patients and their relatives, whilst also helping to initiate conversations regarding goals, expectations and discharge planning.

However, for the ICU patient, their ability to verbally communicate may often be compromised due to the presence of artificial airway devices and respiratory system support [15]. Furthermore, non-verbal communication methods such as gestures or lip-reading are often ineffective and unsuccessful in the ICU due to factors such as weakness or injury [16]. Attempting to communicate via non-verbal methods with ICU patients can subsequently cause frustration, stress and anxiety, for patients, relatives and staff [16].

As well as challenges with communication, history taking from the ICU patient may also be limited by other common factors such as sedation or cognitive impairment [17]. Delirium in the ICU is common and may also be associated with memory impairments, reduced concentration, inattention and poor sleep [18]. Obtaining a detailed and accurate history from the patient in the acute stages of critical illness may therefore be challenging or even impossible, therefore other means may need to be considered.

1.3.2   Taking a History from the Patient's Relatives

Due to the implications of critical illness and ICU therapies, clinicians are often required to collate information from patient relatives. Ideally the clinical team are able to speak with the patients family on a face-to-face consultation, such as during patient visiting hours. This allows the clinician to gauge a sensitive and appropriate time to collate the patient history as part of a natural conversation. Family-centred care and family visitation is advocated by ICU guidelines, with known benefits upon patient outcomes [19–21].

However, coordination of timings between clinicians and visiting times may not always be possible, therefore reliant instead upon telephone communication. Although convenient, it is important to recognise that relatives can experience stress and panic when receiving telephone calls from the hospital when a loved-one is in ICU [22]. It is important to start the telephone call with reassurance and maintain calm and empathetic communication throughout.

There has been significant learning and reflection following the COVID-19 pandemic regarding relative communication. In the height of the pandemic, hospital visiting restrictions were implemented to maintain public safety [23–25]. In addition to the visitation restrictions, telephone communication was also challenging due to face masks and personal protective equipment hampering the ability to hear and speak clearly [23, 26]. This breakdown in family-centred ICU care had profound effects, with moral distress, emotional exhaustion and reduced job satisfaction reported amongst healthcare workers during the COVID-19 pandemic [21, 23, 25, 27].

1.3.3   Video Consultations

To lessen the effect of the COVID-19 quarantine restrictions, guidelines were published to support alternative modes of communications and enable creative and flexible family-centred ICU care [23, 28]. Although unable to replace the value of physical presence at the bedside, video calls offered one alternative [22, 29]. 'Virtual visiting' enabled family members in any geographical locations to connect with the patient. It also allowed the patient to be immersed back into their everyday life and virtually take them to their own home, or to wider members of their support network, including pets [30]. Although there are conflicting perspectives regarding virtual interactions, with care to be taken to adhere to patient consent and privacy, it can continue to offer an alternative method of family communication when in-person visitation is limited [31].

1.3.4   Family Liaison Teams

Another useful communication tool adopted at the height of the COVID-19 pandemic was the use of Family Liaison Teams (FLT). FLT were specialist teams dedicated to relative communication, information and support and were associated with high levels of satisfaction by patient families [24, 32]. In some cases, they also facilitated the 'virtual visiting', bedside photographs, voice recordings or music playlists sent in by relatives [26].

Although visitation is now possible again, the COVID-19 pandemic has reinforced the importance of family members being informed and connected in ICU patient care [29]. Whether in person, by telephone or a virtual platform, attaining a patient history requires a sensitive approach due to the grief, stress and emotion experienced by relatives of ICU patients [9].

It is important that appropriate time is given for retrieving a good history. It may require time and perseverance to gain a detailed understanding of the patient, and clinicians should consider that it is not always possible to gather all information in a single meeting or from one individual. In order to help initiate and structure these conversations, there are tools which may be used to help.

1.3.5   The Clinical Frailty Scale

Frailty, distinct from co-morbidity and age, is a state of vulnerability predisposing certain individuals to increased risk of falls, delirium, disability, and mortality during hospitalization, which consequently increases length of hospitalization stay [33].

Baseline functional status in addition to the burden of pre-existing illness is considered to have prognostic value in the ICU [34]. The development of critical illness may lead to frailty in vulnerable patients; furthermore, critical illness may impede recovery in those already considered frail [35]. Frailty is therefore an important short-term prognostic tool, with frail patients more likely to experience adverse events and have longer lengths of stay in ICU and hospital [36]. Furthermore, in the longer term, frail patients are more likely to leave hospital with impaired functional dependence and quality of life and have greater mortality [36].

The Clinical Frailty Scale (CFS) provides clinicians with an easily applicable tool to stratify according to the level of vulnerability [33]. Although the components of frailty are well known to be complex and diverse, time constraints necessitate a simple assessment tool that is easy to complete on ICU admission, by patients or their relatives [34] (Fig. 1.1). Although the CFS does not provide a detailed history, in the early and acute stages, this may help ICU clinicians to understand the dependency, or independency of their patients, considering health status, physical activity levels and functional participation in activities of daily life. The CFS therefore helps to develop a picture of physical and non-physical risk factors of ICU recovery and may help clinicians to identify their patient's potential rehabilitation and care needs.

1.3.6   Patient Questionnaires: Key Relative Involvement

Documents such as the 'All About Me' or 'This is Me' are commonly used in dementia care and have been adapted for use in the ICU, where patients may not be able to communicate key facts about themselves. These are useful tools when collecting a patient history in the ICU (Fig. 1.2). The questionnaires aim to capture detailed personal information about the patient, including their family and significant others, hobbies, work and independence with activities of daily living. This information is then recorded in a single document accessible for all staff involved in the patient's care. The use of this document, displayed with a photograph, serves as

Clinical Frailty Scale*

 1 **Very Fit** – People who are robust, active, energetic and motivated. These people commonly exercise regularly. They are among the fittest for their age.

 2 **Well** – People who have **no active disease symptoms** but are less fit than category 1. Often, they exercise or are very **active occasionally**, e.g. seasonally.

 3 **Managing Well** – People whose **medical problems are well controlled**, but are **not regularly active** beyond routine walking.

 4 **Vulnerable** – While **not dependent** on others for daily help, often **symptoms limit activities**. A common complaint is being "slowed up", and/or being tired during the day.

 5 **Mildly Frail** – These people often have **more evident slowing**, and need help in **high order IADLs** (finances, transportation, heavy housework, medications). Typically, mild frailty progressively impairs shopping and walking outside alone, meal preparation and housework.

 6 **Moderately Frail** – People need help with **all outside activities** and with **keeping house**. Inside, they often have problems with stairs and need **help with bathing** and might need minimal assistance (cuing, standby) with dressing.

 7 **Severely Frail** – **Completely dependent for personal care**, from whatever cause (physical or cognitive). Even so, they seem stable and not at high risk of dying (within ~ 6 months).

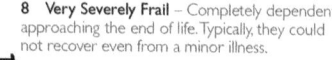 8 **Very Severely Frail** – Completely dependent, approaching the end of life. Typically, they could not recover even from a minor illness.

 9. **Terminally Ill** - Approaching the end of life. This category applies to people with **a life expectancy <6 months**, who are **not otherwise evidently frail**.

Scoring frailty in people with dementia

The degree of frailty corresponds to the degree of dementia. Common **symptoms in mild dementia** include forgetting the details of a recent event, though still remembering the event itself, repeating the same question/story and social withdrawal.

In **moderate dementia**, recent memory is very impaired, even though they seemingly can remember their past life events well. They can do personal care with prompting.

In **severe dementia**, they cannot do personal care without help.

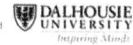 **DALHOUSIE UNIVERSITY** *Inspiring Minds*

Fig. 1.1 Clinical frailty scale. (Reproduced with permission from Dalhousie University)

a reminder of the person who is the patient. The frequent use of prone positioning during the COVID-19 pandemic led to feelings of dehumanised, depersonalised and 'faceless' patient care [25]. A patient photograph can be a valuable way of allowing staff to connect with their patients and knowing the 'person' before they became a patient.

By providing a questionnaire to the family member, it allows them to write down this information in their own time. Considering their stress, emotion and grief, this can often be a more appropriate and sensitive way to collect a good history and can subsequently be a more comfortable approach for healthcare professionals. Relatives commonly report that completing the questionnaire is a therapeutic task, particularly at a time when they feel helpless, valuing the importance of their input in describing the person who has become our patient. It also prevents repetitive conversations for relatives who may come across many different professionals during the course of the patient's ICU admission.

From a clinician's perspective, it is very useful to understand the patient's history from the relatives' perspective, not only knowing their medical and social history but also their likes, dislikes and aspects of their personality. This can help to personalise care and ensure that rehabilitation is patient centred. This can be comforting and reassuring not only for the patient but also their relatives, knowing that their nurse or therapist has taken the time to understand the patient and utilise the 'All About Me' or 'This is Me' to inform *person*-centred care.

THIS IS ME

This information is designed to provide the staff caring for your relative with an insight into who they are – it is hoped that by having a better understanding of a patient's normal environment and lifestyle we can aim to provide aspects of care that are tailored to their individual needs. Please help us by completing the information below and providing a photo of your relative.

Name – Likes to be known as: _____

Insert photo here	
Spiritual/Religious/Cultural beliefs	**Occupation:**
Disability (hearing aid/glasses/walking stick etc.):	**Preferred TV/radio station:**
Interests/hobbies:	**Social – family/friends/pets:**
Any other information (i.e. Right/Left handed, things which may worry or upset me :	

Adapted from www.dignityincare.org.uk/

Fig. 1.2 Example of a 'This is Me' document

1.4   What a Good History Should Include in the ICU

The overall aim of the history is to inform patient-centred care that is respective of and responsive to the individual patient's preferences, needs and values. A good history should therefore consider a holistic overview of the patient's physical, psychological and social needs, as listed in Table 1.1.

Table 1.1 Suggested topics and questions included in a detailed patient history

Topic	Questions to consider
Family	• Who does the patient live with? • Who is their next of kin? • Who is important to the patient? This may include direct family, close friends, neighbours or pets • Do family live locally? If not, will relatives be able to visit? • When are family usually able visit the patient?
Mobility	• Prior to admission could the patient mobilise independently? • Did they require any mobility aids? • Could they manage the stairs? • Were they able to leave the house? • What was their outdoor mobility like? • What was their exercise tolerance like? If limited, why? • Is there any history of falls?
Functional independence and housing	• Can the patient complete all activities of daily living independently? Including washing, dressing, cooking, shopping, cleaning and house-work • Did the patient have any support with any functional activities? • If so, who from? • Did the patient require a package of care or assistance from any carers; do they require social services support? • Are they normally continent? • Where does the patient live? Are they local? • What type of accommodation do they live in? • Are there stairs or steps to access the property? • Is the bedroom and bathroom up or downstairs?
Hobbies, interests and employment	• Did the patient work prior to admission? • If not, when did they stop working and why? • What do/did they do for a living? • What do they like to do in their spare time? • Do they have any hobbies? • Do they follow any sports or teams? • What TV and radio stations do they like? • Do they like to listen to certain music?
Medical issues	• Did the patient have any health problems prior to admission? • How do their health problems affect them? Physically and non-physically including fatigue, mood or pain • How are their health problems managed? • Are they under any specialist medical or support teams? • Have they required ICU or hospital care before? • Were they deconditioned or malnourished pre-admission? • Do they have any mental health issues? • Any history of alcohol, drugs or smoking? • Vaccination status? • Any issues with their vision? Do they wear glasses? • Any issues with their hearing? Do they wear hearing aids?

(continued)

Table 1.1   (continued)

Topic	Questions to consider
Lifestyle	• What is the patient's normal, daily routine? • Do they normally have any issues with sleep? • Do they normally have any issues with pain? • How do they like their appearance? E.g., are they clean shaven? • What is their favourite food or drink?
Understanding and expectations	• What is the patient's perception of their own problems? • What are their main concerns? • Do they understand why these problems have occurred? • What is their expectation of recovery? • What is there understanding of what has happened? • Do they have memory loss? • Do they have insight and understanding?

It is important to ensure that history taking is a caring, empathetic conversation, rather than a checklist, paying due attention to the primary language of the patient and their relatives. History taking requires good communication and active listening skills. The information is personal and important to the patient and their families, as it is these finer details which make the patient a person. It is therefore important to give the patient and their families time to convey this information, showing respect and understanding during the stressful experience of ICU.

1.5   Why an Early, Detailed History Is Important

The rationale for why an early, detailed patient history is necessary and valuable to patient care is detailed below, considering each of the topics outlined in Table 1.1. To appreciate the importance of a history in the ICU, it may be beneficial to consider patient examples.

Patient 1:

A 68-year-old patient has had three failed sedation holds and is now 6 days into her ICU stay following emergency surgery. Staff have recorded that her waking response is neurologically inappropriate and that she is agitated and confused. She is listed for a tracheostomy today and potentially a head CT. A later detailed history from the family reveals the patient normally wears glasses, has bilateral hearing aids and her first language is Urdu. Her glasses and hearing aids were left at home, and the sedation holds were completed without the family present, by English-speaking staff. She is normally very active and independent; she walks to the local library every week and is a member of a book-club.

Patient 2:

An elderly patient is distressed and has pulled out her NG tube. She has remained in bed for the last 5 days as she is restless and considered unsafe to get out of bed. She has required low-dose sedation at night-time and therefore unable to transfer to the ward. Following a detailed history, it is revealed that she has a background of severe arthritis of the hip and requires daily analgesia. Despite her pain, she remains fully independent, living at home alone. She is mobile with a walking-stick and is able to drive, going to the shops and church on a weekly basis. Unfortunately, her usual medication has not been prescribed. She was initially given morphine, yet this was ceased as it caused constipation and nil further analgesia was prescribed. She has not opened her bowels for 2 days.

1.5.1 Family: Key Relationships

Post-traumatic stress after ICU is common amongst patients and their relatives. Involvement of family in the ICU can improve patient care as well as offer support and reassurance to the family themselves [37]. Furthermore, rehabilitation goal setting requires family support and engagement, as recommended by NICE guidelines [4]. In the example of Patient 1, family members could offer support with language interpretation as well as offer reassurance to the patient at a time of fear, disorientation and distress. Knowing who is important to the patient and including them in care can be reassuring and comforting for the patient as well as their relatives. Once Patient 1 had been successfully weaned from sedation, family could also help to support with rehabilitation sessions by offering interpretation or provide incentive to rehabilitation goals. For example, a short-term goal could be for the patient to transfer to the chair for 1 hour periods during relative visiting hours or during a relative video call, to enable social interaction. Photographs and cards from family members could be brought in to the patient's bed-space to make the environment feel less clinical and disorientating. Relatives often feel disempowered and separated from their loved ones and simple involvement in aspects of care reinforces their unique position in progression towards recovery, giving them a valued sense of purpose. Another useful tool to help empower family members in their relatives care is to encourage them to contribute to an ICU patient diary [38, 39]. The ICU diary is a document that the ICU team and families can contribute to on a daily basis. The diary can help patients understand what has happened to them during their admission and fills in the potential gaps in time.

1.5.2 Mobility

Having a good understanding of the patient's baseline level of mobility is important to help set expectations of recovery. This also helps to inform rehabilitation goals, which should be communicated and implemented by all members of the ICU team. For example, Patient 2 may require more intensive rehabilitation due to potential pain, stiffness and weakness associated with arthritis in addition to bed rest and critical illness. In this instance, the nurses could help Patient 2 into the chair for her breakfast and encourage her to participate in her own wash, then later the physiotherapy team could review to practice mobilisation with a frame and complete a strengthening exercise programme. Involving all members of the team helps to promote a normal daily routine for the patient and also provides consistency to care and rehabilitation. Understanding the patient's history and baseline mobility at an early stage may also help to inform the care and rehabilitation needs of the patient beyond ICU discharge.

In the example of Patient 2, it may be necessary to consider early referral to specialist teams, such as pain management, pharmacy or orthopaedic teams.

1.5.3   Functional Status and Housing

Understanding the patient's previous levels of functional independence may also help to guide the level of support a patient may need during their ICU and hospital stay. If previously independent, ICU clinicians should consider engaging patients in appropriate functional tasks and setting functional goals, as clinically appropriate. For example, can the patient participate in their own wash rather than have a passive bed-bath, or can they sit out of bed for meal times and feed themselves? This helps to empower patients in their care and recovery, which in turn provides a normal daily routine to try improve their sleep and orientation.

Furthermore, understanding the patient's history may help to identify if occupational therapy or social care referrals can be made. For example, if the patient previously lived in a third floor flat and was struggling to manage at home alone, then they may require increased support on ICU discharge. Anticipating the needs of the patient during acute ICU care enhances timely organisation and coordination of resources and provides time to develop discharge plans [3].

1.5.4   Hobbies, Interests and Work

Personalising care and rehabilitation is important in the ICU, particularly when patients may be fatigued, scared or low in mood and motivation. Engaging with the patient on a meaningful and personal level may offer them reassurance, motivation, hope or distraction. It may also offer a way for relatives to engage with the patient, such as watching a television programme together or playing their favourite music. For example, Patient 1 could be encouraged to read when awake during day-time hours, have photographs of her family at her bedside or a communication chart written in Urdu. Overall, understanding the patient can help to make care personal, tolerable and interactive for ICU patients, relatives and staff.

1.5.5   Medical History

An understanding of the patient's medical history is not only important to guide medical management but to also appreciate their level of dependency and frailty. This may help to guide the ICU clinicians' expectations of recovery and set appropriate goals and expectations with relatives necessary to guide discharge planning. In contrast, it is important to understand the full effects and consequences of the patient's history without assumptions. Despite initial expectations of being elderly, frail and delirious, Patient 1 required her hearing aids, glasses and an interpreter whilst Patient 2 required appropriate pain and bowel management.

1.5.6   Lifestyle History

A detailed history also helps to understand the individual person to inform person-alised care. In the hospital environment, we often enforce our routine upon the patient, coordinating patient care around meal times, staff breaks, drug administra-tion or ward rounds. However, if pre-admission the patient had difficulties with sleep or worked night shifts for example, it is reasonable to expect that the patient may have difficulties with sleep and routine in the ICU. Understanding the patients normal routine may also help to inform rehabilitation and offer guidance for goal setting. For example, Patient 1 may wish to have mobility goals focused on walking to the book-club or Patient 2 may wish to be able to go to the hospitals chaplaincy service. Furthermore, supporting patients with functional day-to-day tasks is impor-tant, such as getting dressed in their own clothes or being able to comb their hair. This may help the patient to feel 'human', rather than a dependent ICU patient.

1.5.7   Understanding and Expectations

Developing an understanding of the patient's perceptions, beliefs and expectations is important to guide care and communication. If the patient lacks insight and under-standing, perhaps due to common factors such as memory loss, sedation or delir-ium, this may confound their reasoning and capacity to make appropriate decisions. It may help clinicians to inform and educate patients on the expectations of recovery and the common symptoms of critical illness. This may help patients and relatives to be more engaged in their recovery.

1.6   Conclusions

Retrieving a patient history in the ICU can be challenging, but with a sensitive and structured approach, it enables clinicians to develop therapeutic relationships with patients and their relatives. A detailed understanding of the patient subsequently helps to establish meaningful and appropriate rehabilitation goals, aiming to over-come the physical and non-physical consequences of critical illness. The patient history also allows clinicians to understand their patients as an individual, providing compassionate care that considers the patient's holistic needs. Ultimately this aims to improve patient outcomes, not only as a *patient* overcoming critical illness but empowering the individual in their recovery to the *person*.

Key Take Home Messages

- Aim to obtain a detailed history as soon as possible and appropriate following ICU admission, ensuring that the timing is sensitive to the clinical situation.
- Utilise the information obtained to set meaningful, appropriate and patient-centred rehabilitation goals with the patient and their relatives.

- Deliver compassionate and sensitive care ensuring that the patient's individual needs, values, likes and dislikes are taken into account.
- Make multidisciplinary team referrals early to prevent delay in patient care.
- Ensure communication between the team and the patient and their family is sustained throughout their entire admission.

References

1. Backes MT, Erdmann AL, Büscher A. The living, dynamic and complex environment care in intensive care unit. Rev Lat Am Enfermagem. 2015;23(3):411–8. https://doi.org/10.1590/0104-1169.0568.2570.
2. Merilainen M, Kyngas H, Ala-Kokko T. 24-Hour intensive care: an observational study of an environment and events. Intensive Crit Care Nurs. 2010;26(5):246–53.
3. Holland DE, Rhudy LM, Vanderboom CE, Bowles KH. Feasibility of discharge planning in intensive care units: a pilot study. Am J Crit Care. 2012;21(4):e94–e101. https://doi.org/10.4037/ajcc2012173.
4. National Institute for Health and Care Excellence. Rehabilitation after critical illness in adults clinical guideline CG83. 2009. nice.org.uk/guidance/cg83.
5. Rawal G, Yadav S, Kumar R. Post-intensive care syndrome: an overview. J Transl Int Med. 2017;5(2):90–2. https://doi.org/10.1515/jtim-2016-0016.
6. Herridge MS, Tansey CM, Matte A, et al. Functional disability 5 years after acute respiratory distress syndrome. N Engl J Med. 2011;364(14):1293–304.
7. Fromage G. Medical records and history taking. J Aesthet Nurs. 2018;7(10):538–40. https://doi.org/10.12968/joan.2018.7.10.538.
8. Lloyd C. A guide to taking a patient's history. Nurs Stand. 2007;22(13):42–8.
9. Anderson WG, Arnold RM, Angus DC, et al. Posttraumatic stress and complicated grief in family members of patients in the intensive care unit. J Gen Intern Med. 2008;23(11):1871–6. https://doi.org/10.1007/s11606-008-0770-2.
10. Farahani MA, Gaeeni M, Mohammadi N, Seyedfatemi N. Giving information to family members of patients in the intensive care unit: Iranian nurses' ethical approaches. J Med Ethics Hist Med. 2014;7:9.
11. Pochard FF, Azoulay FE, Chevert FS, Lemaire FF, Hubert FP, Canoui FP, Grassin FM, Zittoun FR, Le Gall FJR, Dhainaut FJ, Schlemmer FB. Symptoms of anxiety and depression in family members of the intensive care unit patients: ethical hypothesis regarding decision-making capacity. Crit Care Med. 2001;29(10):1893–7.
12. Jones C, Skirrow P, Griffiths R, Humphris G, Ingleby S, Eddleston J, Waldmann C, Gager M. Post-traumatic stress disorder-related symptoms in relatives of patients following intensive care. Intensive Care Med. 2004;30(3):456–60. https://doi.org/10.1007/s00134-003-2149-5.
13. National Institute for Health and Care Excellence. Rehabilitation after critical illness in adults Quality Standard QS158. 2017. https://www.nice.org.uk/guidance/qs158/resources/rehabilitation-after-critical-illness-in-adults-pdf-75545546693317.
14. Bovend'Eerdt T, Botell R, Wade D. Writing SMART rehabilitation goals and achieving goal attainment scaling: a practical guide. Clin Rehabil. 2009;23:352–61.
15. Rotondi AJ, Chelluri LR, Sirio CR, Mendelsohn AR, Schulz RR, Belle SR, Im RK, Donahoe MR, Pinsky MR. Patients recollections of stressful experiences while receiving prolonged mechanical ventilation in an intensive care unit. Crit Care Med. 2002;30(4):746–52.
16. ten Hoorn S, Elbers PW, Girbes AR, Tuinman PR. Communicating with conscious and mechanically ventilated critically ill patients: a systematic review. Crit Care. 2016;20(1):333. https://doi.org/10.1186/s13054-016-1483-2.

17. Wade DM, Howell DC, Weinman JA, Hardy RJ, Mythen MG, Brewin CR, et al. Investigating risk factors for psychological morbidity three months after intensive care: a prospective cohort study. Crit Care. 2012;16(5):R192.

18. Balas MC, Weinhouse GL, Denehy L, Chanques G, Rochwerg B, Misak CJ, et al. Interpreting and implementing the 2018 pain, agitation/sedation, delirium, immobility, and sleep disruption clinical practice guideline. Crit Care Med. 2018;46(9):1464–70.

19. Davidson JE, Aslakson RA, Long AC, et al. Guidelines for family-centered care in the neonatal, pediatric, and adult ICU. Crit Care Med. 2017;45(1):103–28. https://doi.org/10.1097/CCM.0000000000002169.

20. Ely EW. The ABCDEF Bundle: science and philosophy of how ICU liberation serves patients and families. Crit Care Med. 2017;45(2):321–30. https://doi.org/10.1097/CCM.0000000000002175.

21. Azoulay É, Curtis JR, Kentish-Barnes N. Ten reasons for focusing on the care we provide for family members of critically ill patients with COVID-19. Intensive Care Med. 2021;47:230–3. https://doi.org/10.1007/s00134-020-06319-.

22. Forsberg T, Isaksson M, Schelin C, Lyngå P, Schandl A. Family members' experiences of COVID-19 visiting restrictions in the intensive care unit—a qualitative study. J Clin Nurs. 2023;33:215–23. https://doi.org/10.1111/jocn.16637.

23. Hart JL, Turnbull AE, Oppenheim IM, Courtright KR. Family-centered care during the COVID-19 era. J Pain Symptom Manag. 2020;60(2):e93–7. https://doi.org/10.1016/j.jpainsymman.2020.04.017.

24. Lopez-Soto C, Bates E, Anderson C, et al. The role of a liaison team in ICU family communication during the COVID 19 pandemic. J Pain Symptom Manag. 2021;62(3):e112–9. https://doi.org/10.1016/j.jpainsymman.2021.04.008.

25. Eskell M, Thompson J, Powell O, Torlinski T, Mullhi R. Understanding the intensive care unit experience of patients and relatives at the end-of-life during the coronavirus disease 2019 pandemic. J Patient Exp. 2022;9:23743735221106586. https://doi.org/10.1177/23743735221106586.

26. Baker L, Lindsay H, Payton-Crisp C, et al. 12 isolated but not alone: critical care communication in the time of covid-19. BMJ Leader. 2020;4:A4–5. https://doi.org/10.1136/leader-2020-FMLM.12.

27. McPeake J, Kentish-Barnes N, Banse E, et al. Clinician perceptions of the impact of ICU family visiting restrictions during the COVID-19 pandemic: an international investigation. Crit Care. 2023;27(1):33. https://doi.org/10.1186/s13054-023-04318-8.

28. Intensive Care Society. ICS guidance on the use of video communication for patients and relatives in ICU. https://www.acprc.org.uk/Data/Resource_Downloads/Covid19_ICSGuidanceontheuseofvideocommunucationforpatientsandrelative....pdf?date=28/06/2020%2015:09:45202028/06/2020%2015:09:452020. Accessed 19 May 2023.

29. Chen C, Wittenberg E, Sullivan SS, Lorenz RA, Chang YP. The experiences of family members of ventilated COVID-19 patients in the intensive care unit: a qualitative study. Am J Hosp Palliat Care. 2021;38(7):869–76. https://doi.org/10.1177/10499091211006914.

30. Xyrichis A, Pattison N, Ramsay P, et al. Virtual visiting in intensive care during the COVID-19 pandemic: a qualitative descriptive study with ICU clinicians and non-ICU family team liaison members. BMJ Open. 2022;12:e055679. https://doi.org/10.1136/bmjopen-2021-055679.

31. Kennedy NR, Steinberg A, Arnold RM, Doshi AA, White DB, DeLair W, Nigra K, Elmer J. Perspective on telephone and video communication in the intensive care unit during COVID-19. Ann Am Thorac Soc. 2021;18(5):838–47. https://doi.org/10.1513/AnnalsATS.202006-729OC.

32. Klop HT, Nasori M, Klinge TW, et al. Family support on intensive care units during the COVID-19 pandemic: a qualitative evaluation study into experiences of relatives. BMC Health Serv Res. 2021;21:1060. https://doi.org/10.1186/s12913-021-07095-8.

33. Juma S, Taabazuing MM, Montero-Odasso M. Clinical Frailty Scale in an acute medicine unit: a simple tool that predicts length of stay. Can Geriatr J 2016;19(2):34–9. https://doi.org/10.5770/cgj.19.196. https://www.ncbi.nlm.nih.gov/pmc/articles/PMC4922366..

34. McDermid R, Stelfox H, Bagshaw S. Frailty in the critically ill: a novel concept. Crit Care. 2011;15:301.

35. Muscedere J, Waters B, Varambally A, Bagshaw SM, Boyd JG, Maslove D, et al. The impact of frailty on intensive care unit outcomes: a systematic review and meta-analysis. Intensive Care Med. 2017;43(8):1105–22. https://doi.org/10.1007/s00134-017-4867-0.

36. Bagshaw S, Stelfox T, McDermid R, Rolfson D, Tsuyuki R, Baig N, Artiuch B, Ibrahim Q, Stollery D, Rokosh E, Majumdar S. Association between frailty and short- and long-term outcomes among critically ill patients: a multicentre prospective cohort study. Can Med Assoc J. 2014;186(2):E95–E102. https://doi.org/10.1503/cmaj.130639.

37. Wyskiel R, Weeks K, Marsteller J. Inviting families to participate in care: a family involvement in menu. Jt Comm J Qual Patient Saf. 2015;41(1):43–6. https://doi.org/10.1016/S1553-7250(15)41006-2.

38. Rice RN, Qualls BW, Carey MG. Use of diaries for family members of intensive care unit patients to reduce long-term PTSD: a pilot study. J Patient Exp. 2022;9:23743735221105681. https://doi.org/10.1177/23743735221105681.

39. Mickelson RS, Piras SE, Brown L, Carlile C, Drumright KS, Boehm L. The use and usefulness of ICU diaries to support family members of critically ill patients. J Crit Care. 2021;61:168–76. https://doi.org/10.1016/j.jcrc.2020.10.003.

Respiratory and Mechanical Ventilation Management: Avoidance of Complications

2

Roberto Martinez-Alejos, Ricardo Miguel Rodrigues-Gomes, and Joan-Daniel Martí

2.1 Introduction

Critically ill patients receiving invasive mechanical ventilation (IMV) often present with impaired airway clearance resulting in retention of airway secretions [1]. Consequently, excessive accumulation of secretions within the respiratory system and artificial airways increases airflow resistance and work of breathing, causes breathing discomfort and may slow ventilator weaning [2, 3]. Moreover, mucus retained within peripheral airways, which cannot be removed through suctioning, may also lead to airway collapse and hinder gas exchange.

Several factors have been associated with mucus retention in the critically ill (Fig. 2.1) with endotracheal intubation considered as the primary mechanism. Indeed, mucociliary clearance rates may be reduced by as much as 80% after intubation and inflation of the endotracheal tube (ETT) cuff [4]. This is caused by the addition of positive pressure and PEEP, along with a presumed decrease in perfusion of the tracheal mucosa and/or a response of the sympathetic nervous system caused by the cuff. In addition, the inflated ETT cuff exerts a mechanical barrier that impedes clearance of airway secretions reaching the proximal trachea; thus, causing mucus to accumulate in this region if the patient is unable to expectorate and/or suction is not performed. Nevertheless, recurrent airway suctioning may be necessary as the procedure is limited to the first bronchial division, resulting in an increased

R. Martinez-Alejos (✉)
Montpellier Trainning School of Physiotherapy, Montpellier, France

Kernel Biomedical, Bois-Guillaume, France

R. M. Rodrigues-Gomes
Intensive Care Unit, Hospital Álvaro Cunqueiro, Vigo, Spain

J.-D. Martí
Cardiovascular Surgery ICU, Hospital Clinic, Barcelona, Spain

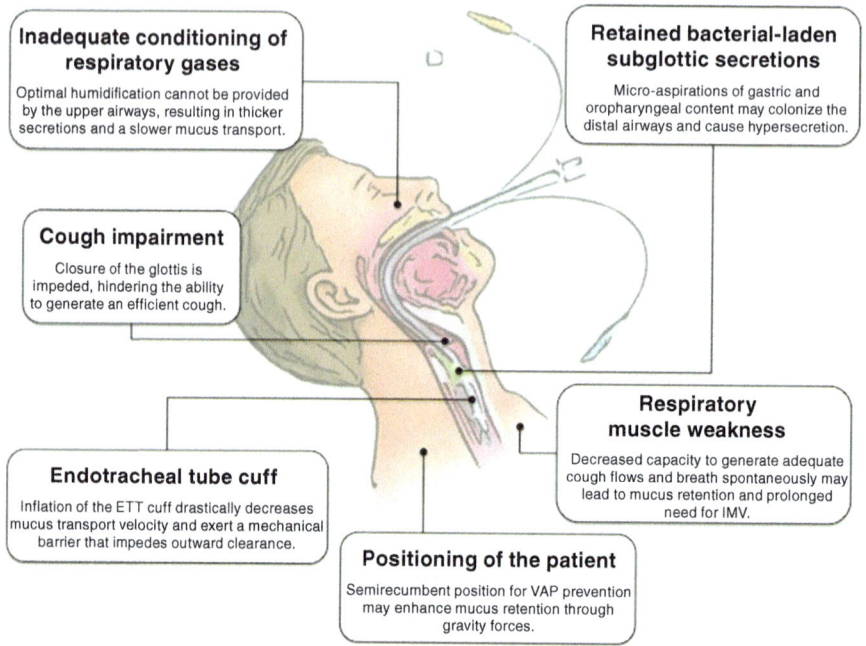

Fig. 2.1 Main causes of mucus retention in the critically ill on invasive mechanical ventilation. *ETT* endotracheal tube, *IMV* invasive mechanical ventilation

risk for damage to the tracheal mucosa, oxygen desaturation and airway collapse. Additionally, cough efficacy is highly impaired in the intubated patient as the presence of an ETT within the trachea obstructs the closure of the glottis [5].

Under normal conditions, upper airways provide up to 75% of the absolute humidity necessary to ensure adequate functioning of the alveolar–capillary interface (i.e. 44 mgH$_2$O/L of air). Of note, optimal absolute humidity requires relative moisture of 100% at 37 °C of temperature. However, during IMV, the upper airways are bypassed by the artificial airway and optimal conditioning of the respiratory gases is impeded. Inadequate humidification, even for short periods, impairs cilia function and damages the airway epithelium, resulting in thicker secretions and decreased mucus transport velocity [6]. Thus, the use of electro-mechanical devices (e.g. heated humidifiers) or filters (e.g. heat and moisture exchangers) that supply heat and moisture is mandatory to optimise conditioning of the delivered ventilation.

Retained respiratory secretions often become colonised, increasing the risk of developing lung infections [7]. When present, respiratory infections may impair the cilia function, further enhancing the production of respiratory secretions and altering mucus properties. Moreover, continuous leakage of bacteria-laden subglottic secretions around the ETT cuff may eventually colonise the lower airways in the intubated patients [8], especially when enterally fed. Although still of significant controversy, translocation of pathogens from oropharyngeal and gastric content to the distal lung parenchyma has been suggested as the principle mechanism for ventilator-associated pneumonia (VAP) [9, 10]. Hence, suctioning of subglottic content and positioning of the patient in the semi-recumbent position are strategies commonly implemented in the intensive care unit (ICU) to prevent such complications [11]. Of note, placing the patients supine with the head of the bed elevated 30–45° above the horizontal (i.e. semi-recumbent position) is recommended to reduce gastroesophageal reflux and, consequently, the risk for VAP. However, during this position, retention of airway secretions may be enhanced by gravity forces and mucus moves towards and into the lungs [12].

Critically ill patients are often confined to prolonged periods of bed rest due to clinical instability, complex care needs (e.g. central extracorporeal membrane oxygenation), or logistical barriers. It is well known that immobility and ICU-acquired polyneuromyopathy [13] leads to the development of moderate to severe muscular deconditioning and physical functioning impairment, resulting in a prolonged need for ICU and hospital stay [14]. Limb muscle weakness has been correlated with respiratory muscle impairment in these patients, affecting cough efficacy and delaying weaning from mechanical ventilation [15]. Additionally, diaphragmatic function and force may also be affected during mechanical ventilation as the muscle activity is reduced or, especially in controlled modes, completely suppressed. Indeed, ventilator-induced diaphragmatic dysfunction [16] is highly prevalent even after short periods of mechanical ventilation and has been associated with increased weaning periods, and hospital/ICU mortality. Although there is still a paucity of robust evidence, several studies reported early physiotherapy and mobilisation as a feasible and safe strategy to improve muscular and functional outcomes in the critically ill and to reduce the need for IMV and hospital/ICU length of stay [17]. Furthermore, promising results from a growing body of evidence suggest respiratory muscle training as a potential intervention to improve weaning outcomes in selected population of patients [18–21].

2.2 Respiratory Management During Invasive Mechanical Ventilation

2.2.1 Endotracheal Suctioning

Endotracheal suctioning (ETS) is commonly performed in the critically ill as the principal strategy to remove bronchial secretions and ensure patency of the artificial airway [22]. Although this procedure has no absolute contraindications, ETS is not exempt from associated risks and complications such as oxygen desaturation, damage of the tracheal/bronchial mucosa, lung de-recruitment or respiratory infections. Also the efficacy of the manoeuvre is often limited to the tracheal carina and, consequently, the need for repetitive suctioning may further enhance the risk of complications. Performing ETS following current recommendations [22] is strongly suggested to avoid associated detrimental effects and ensure the safety of the procedure (Table 2.1). Importantly, the aforementioned recommendations do not consider

Table 2.1 Recommendations for endotracheal suctioning in critically ill patients on invasive mechanical ventilation

Recommendations

• Endotracheal suctioning should be performed only when secretions are present, and not routinely
    – ETS at least every 8 h has been suggested to avoid partial occlusion of the artificial airway
    – The main clinical indicators for mucus retention in the intubated and mechanically ventilated patients are the presence of a 'sawtooth' pattern in the expiratory phase of the flow-volume curve of the ventilator [22, 23], the presence of coarse crackles over the trachea and/or visual secretions within the artificial airway

• Pre-oxygenation should be considered if the patient has a clinically important reduction in oxygen saturation with suctioning
    – The delivery of 100% oxygen for at least 30–60 s before and after the procedure is recommended to avoid ETS-induced hypoxemia
    – It is recommended to enrich oxygen delivery by manually adjusting the F_IO_2 or through dedicated software of the ventilators rather than using manual ventilations through a resuscitator bag

• Performing suctioning without disconnecting the patient from the ventilator is suggested

• Use of shallow suction is suggested instead of deep suction
    – Shallow suctioning (up to the distal tip of the artificial airway or the tracheal carina) is preferred to deep suctioning to prevent mucosal trauma or pulmonary collapse (evidence based on paediatric population)
    – Importantly, the depth of suctioning must be adapted depending on the artificial airway that is used (i.e.: endotracheal or tracheostomy tube)

• It is suggested that routine use of normal saline instillation prior to endotracheal suction should not be performed
    – Normal saline instillation is commonly used to facilitate the outward clearance of thick secretions
    – Instillation of saline may result in negative outcomes such as patient discomfort, oxygen desaturation, airway spasm, and translocation of pathogens present within the artificial airway to the lower airways
    – Of note, evidence from a single randomised control trial associated instillation of normal saline before suctioning with a significant reduction of microbiological proven VAP when compared to no instillation [24]

• Closed and open suctioning can be indistinctively used as both systems are sage and effective in paediatric and adult patients. Of note, open suctioning must be performed using a sterile technique

• It is suggested that the suction catheter used should occludes less than 50% of the lumen of the ETT in paediatric and adult patients, and less than 70% in neonatal patients
    – The adequate selection of the suction catheter size (i.e.: external diameter) is a paramount concern to avoid the risk of pulmonary collapse
    – Larger diameter catheters increase the percentage of obstruction in relation to the artificial airway and, consequently, the negative pressure transmitted to the airways
    – Suction pressure should be lower than −200 mmHg in adult patients, and lower than −120 mmHg in neonatal and paediatric patients

• It is suggested that the duration of the suctioning event should be limited to less than 15 s
• Use of bronchoscopy as routine technique to remove secretions is not recommended
• Scraping devices aiming to clear inner diameter of the artificial airways may be used in cases where secretions are cumulated and causing an increase of peak inspiratory pressure and airway resistances

(continued)

Table 2.1 (continued)

Adapted from "Blakeman TC, Scott JB, Yoder MA, Capellari E, Strickland SL. AARC Clinical Practice Guidelines: Artificial Airway Suctioning. Respir Care. 2022 Feb;67(2):258–271" [22]

ETS endotracheal suctioning, F_iO_2 fraction of inspired oxygen, *ETT* endotracheal tube, *mmHg* milimetres of mercury

COVID-19 patients, and the use of closed suction systems to prevent patient and patient to staff cross contamination is strongly recommended in these patients [25].

2.2.2 Subglottic Suctioning

Although the ETT cuff aims to seal the trachea and prevent leakage of fluids accumulated above the cuff, continuous micro-aspiration of subglottic bacterial-laden content is not fully impeded, increasing the risk for distal airways colonisation. The suctioning of oropharyngeal and gastric fluids accrued at the subglottic region may reduce hydrostatic pressure over the ETT cuff and eventually prevent micro-aspiration [26]. Thus, current international guidelines strongly recommend subglottic suctioning as a strategy for VAP prevention [11]. This is performed through a dedicated suction port placed proximally above the cuff of some ETT and tracheostomy tubes. The subglottic port can be connected to a vacuum system or a syringe, and suction is performed continuously or intermittently with no significant differences reported in the literature. Importantly some studies described damage to the tracheal mucosa resulting from the negative pressure transmitted to a specific region of the trachea but the clinical consequences of this damage remain unclear. Hence, it is recommended to perform subglottic suctioning through low-vacuum pressure (100–150 mmHg) [27] or gently pulling back the plunger of the syringe. Additionally, if the suction port is obstructed or blocked (e.g. the backward movement of the plunger is limited), a gentle instillation of 10 mL of air or normal saline is suggested to unstick the suction port from the mucosa.

2.2.3 Humidification of Respiratory Gases

Invasive mechanical ventilation implies the use of an artificial airway (i.e. endotracheal and tracheostomy tube) to transport respiratory gases from the ventilator to the lungs. The delivered airflows enter the lungs approximately at 2–5 cm before the first bronchial division, where the distal tip of the artificial airway is placed. Consequently, upper airways are bypassed, impeding the delivery of the heat and moisture necessary for the alveolar–capillary interface (i.e. absolute humidity of 44 mgH$_2$O/L). Humidification of respiratory gases below 30 mgH$_2$O/L for ≥24 h has been associated with malfunctioning of the airway mucosa; hence, current recommendations advise the provision of a minimum of 30–33 mgH$_2$O/L in patients with artificial airways. Supplemental heat and moisture can be procured passively or actively, through heat and moisture exchanger (HME) filters or heated humidifiers (HH), respectively (Table 2.2) [28].

Evidence comparing the effects of HME and HH in major outcomes such as artificial airway narrowing/occlusion, pneumonia or mortality is contradictory and still inconclusive [29]. However, it is suggested to change HME filters at least every 24–48 h to reduce the likelihood of artificial airway occlusion. Similarly, contradictory results in terms of VAP prevention have been reported in different systematic reviews and meta-analysis comparing both passive and active humidification [29]. Nevertheless, hydrophobic filters may reduce the risk of VAP when compared to hygroscopic HMEs and HH. Finally, as stated by current guidelines recommendations [28], the use of HME may be contraindicated in specific clinical scenarios (Table 2.3).

2.3 Chest Physiotherapy

Chest physiotherapy (CPT) includes a wide range of manual and mechanical techniques intended to facilitate displacement of mucus towards the trachea and to enhance cough efficacy. Thus, CPT is considered an intervention to be implemented when retention of mucus occurs (e.g. the presence of a 'sawtooth' pattern in the flow-volume curve of the ventilator and/or coarse crackles over the trachea) [30]. CPT is also commonly implemented with the aim to improve oxygenation and/or pulmonary mechanics and decrease the incidence of pulmonary infections. Historically, CPT has aimed to improve airway clearance by placing the patient into specific positions that theoretically displace mucus through gravitational forces (i.e. postural drainage). Additionally, positioning was often combined with manual chest

Table 2.2 Humidification systems

Heat and moisture exchanger filters (HME)
• HME filters are placed between the Y-piece of the ventilator circuit and the artificial airway to store heat and moisture exhaled from the patient, to be delivered during the following inspiration
• Filters can be grouped in hydrophobic, which retains temperature and repel moisture between the filter and the patient, and hygroscopic, which are covered with products that absorb water vapor (e.g. calcium chloride)
• HME filters are suggested for patients ventilated <96 h, provided that the system is able to deliver ≥30 mgH$_2$O/L, relative humidity of 100%, and a minimum of 34 °C of temperature for an optimal performance [28]
Heated humidifiers (HH)
• HH actively increase temperature and humidification through the passage of the inspired respiratory gases within a heated water reservoir placed along the inspiratory circuit of the ventilator
• HH should provide absolute humidity of 34–44 mgH$_2$O/L by delivering relative humidity of 100% and gas temperature between 34 and 41 °C [28]
• HH can be complemented by heated-wire circuits aimed to prevent water condensation by maintaining the temperature between the water reservoir and the Y-piece of the ventilator circuit

Table 2.3 Contraindications for the use of heat and moisture exchanger filters

Clinical scenario	Rationale
• Patients with frank bloody or thick, copious secretions	• Increased risk for filter obstruction or augmented resistance to airflow
• Expired tidal volume less than 70% of the delivered tidal volume (e.g. tracheal tube cuff malfunction)	• Sufficient heat and moisture may not reach the filter to ensure its adequate functioning
• Lung-protective ventilation or low delivered tidal volumes	• Volume and positioning of HME devices contribute to additional dead space
• Body temperatures <32 °C	• Sufficient heat may not reach the filter to ensure its adequate functioning
• Hypercapnic patients	• HME may increase the risk for P_aCO_2 retention due to the associated dead space

Adapted from "AARC Clinical Practice Guideline. Humidification during invasive and noninvasive mechanical ventilation: 2012. Respir Care 2012; 57: 782–788"
HME heat and moisture exchanger filter, P_aCO_2 arterial partial pressure of carbon dioxide

percussions (i.e. clapping) or vibrations to stimulate ciliary beating. However, evidence to support the use of these techniques is scarce and controversial [31]. Consequently, chest physiotherapy has evolved into techniques intended to enhance mucus clearance through the modulation of airflows [32]. Indeed, several in vivo [33] and in vitro [32–36] studies have demonstrated that airflows interact with the mucus layer, and airway secretions can be transported towards the lungs or the glottis through the two-phase gas–liquid flow mechanism. Thus, outward mucus clearance may be enhanced when expiratory flow sufficiently exceeds inspiratory flow [36]. A growing body of research corroborates that the most implemented CPT techniques nowadays are manual/ventilator pulmonary hyperinflations and manual chest compressions/vibrations [32]. Additionally, very recent studies have evaluated mechanical in-exsufflation as a potential strategy to improve cough efficacy in intubated and mechanically ventilated patients.

2.3.1 Manual or Ventilator Pulmonary Hyperinflation

Pulmonary hyperinflation is aimed to generate an inspiratory volume higher than tidal volume to improve the clearance of proximal secretions, oxygenation and pulmonary mechanics in patients invasively ventilated. Hyperinflation is achieved manually, through a resuscitator bag, or via modification of the ventilator parameters The technique includes three differentiated phases to achieve the aforementioned objectives: (1) slow delivery (i.e. ≥3 s) of a tidal volume around 50% higher than baseline or until an airway pressure of 40 cmH₂O is reached; (2) inspiratory hold of approximately 3 s to ensure homogeneous distribution of air within the lungs; and (3) prompt release of the pressure to facilitate a rapid pulmonary recoil that enhance expiratory flows [37]. Thus, emphasis in phase 1 and 2 or phase 3 aims to improve, respectively, oxygenation and pulmonary mechanics or mucus clearance. Manual hyperinflation (MHI) and/or ventilator hyperinflation (VHI) are the most studied techniques in critically ill patients along the last two decades. MHI has been associated with significant improvements in compliance on post-cardiac surgery patients, and patients with pneumonia or atelectasis [38], whereas results from studies assessing the effects of MHI on oxygenation are controversial [38]. On the other hand, evidence on MHI to clear airway secretions is overall encouraging, particularly when combined to positioning of the patient in side-laying or head-down tilt and manual chest compressions. Of note, no clinically significant adverse events during MHI have been reported. To date, only few studies compared MHI and VHI with no reported relevant differences between both modalities [38, 39]. It is important to emphasise that the methodology used to implement both MHI and VHI is highly heterogeneous along the available evidence; hence, drawing up robust conclusions is difficult. Indeed, (1) tidal volume and airway pressure are used as a target indistinctly; (2) the time to achieve the target volume/pressure varies from 1 to 4 s and, consequently, inspiratory flow velocity is variable; (3) inspiratory pause and/or rapid pressure release are not always procured; and (4) the number of sessions implemented varies from 2 to 6 sets of 5–10 hyperinflations. As suggested recently by Volpe et al., VHI should be performed in Volume Control Continuous Mandatory Ventilation to achieve an inspiratory flow of 20–40 L/min with the purpose of improve flow bias, generating a difference between Peak Inspiratory Flow and the Peak Expiratory Flow higher than 33 L/m favouring PEF [39].

Several considerations must be taken into account when choosing the best modality to implement pulmonary hyperinflation. MHI implies the disconnection of the patient from the ventilator, resulting in an increased risk for oxygen desaturation and/or lung de-recruitment. Moreover, airway pressures achieved during MHI may be extremely heterogeneous depending on the experience of the practitioner. In-line manometers during MHI or a safety pressure valve (40 cmH_2O) are strongly recommended. Conversely, VHI ensures homogeneous implementation of the procedure and continuous monitoring, without need for disconnection from the ventilator. Therefore, VHI is suggested to be a safer alternative to MHI in the critically ill on IMV, particularly when an elevated respiratory support is required [40].This is particularly the case for those patients with COVID-19 or severe ARDS, where disconnection of the ventilator circuit would increase the risk of infection amongst healthcare staff or patients in adjacent areas. In addition, the ability to more closely monitor peak airway pressures during VHI would be advantageous to minimise the risk of exacerbating acute lung injury in those patients receiving lung protective ventilation. High peak, plateau or driving pressures at baseline may make this difficult or indeed impossible to achieve in those with severe ARDS/COVID-19.

2.3.2 Manual Chest Compressions/Vibrations (MCC)

Manual chest compressions are intended to enhance outward clearance of mucus by exerting manual compressions over the rib cage during exhalation to modulate expiratory flows [41]. Although several different variants of the technique have been proposed in the literature, manual chest compressions can be assembled in two groups dependant on the targeted airways to be cleared. Prompt and strong compressions at very early exhalation are intended to mimic cough and improve mucus clearance from proximal airways by enhancing expiratory peak flow bias. On the other hand, prolonged and gentle compressions during the mid-late expiratory phase are aimed to extend flow–mucus interaction and dislodge secretions from the distal airways such as the prolonged expiratory technique in infants. Although a growing body of clinical evidence has been published along the last decade, the efficacy of MCC in clearing airway secretions is still controversial, mainly due to the heterogeneous implementation of the technique [41]. Slow and soft compressions failed to show any relevant effects on mucus clearance even when combined with side-lying, whereas brief and strong compressions have been associated with improved but not significant outward clearance of airway secretions [42]. Interestingly, results from animal studies reported a significant improvement in mucus displacement (i.e. radiopaque mucus tracking) [43, 44] and mucus weight during hard and brief MCC but without any impact in gas exchange. Conversely, soft and prolonged MCC did not exert any relevant effects on mucus clearance, and adverse effects such as decreased cardiac output and lung compliance were associated with the technique [44]. Thus, since the increase in transthoracic pressure may hinder venous return and increase the risk for airway collapsibility, special attention should be paid during manual chest compressions.

2.4   Mechanical In-Exsufflation (MI-E)

MI-E aims to create high expiratory flow rates to move secretions from the proximal airways towards the trachea for suctioning or expectoration. The technique is implemented through a dedicated electro-mechanical device that gradually applies a positive pressure to the airway and then rapidly shifts to a negative pressure to simulate cough [45]. MI-E is considered the *Gold Standard* technique to improve mucus clearance in neuromuscular patients unable to produce an efficient cough, with associated positive outcomes on the literature. Moreover, the technique can be implemented through a facemask, mouthpiece or an artificial airway; thus, MI-E is nowadays suggested as a potential strategy to enhance peak expiratory cough flows in intubated and mechanically ventilated patients. Very recently, a few studies have evaluated the efficacy and/or safety of MI-E in sedated critically ill patients on IMV, overall reporting promising results [46–48]. Indeed, although notable methodological limitations of the published studies (e.g. use of visual inspection of airway secretions within the ETT to assess the efficacy of the technique), MI-E resulted in improved mucus clearance and a short-term improvement in lung compliance when compared to standard care (i.e. endotracheal suctioning) or a combination of respiratory physiotherapy techniques. Moreover, no clinical significant adverse events were associated with the use of MI-E [46–48].

Since the setting of the device notably varies along with the literature, further research is warranted to elucidate the role and adequate implementation of MI-E. For instance, insufflation–exsufflation pressures of $+40/-40$ cmH$_2$O are suggested to be the most comfortable and effective setting in neuromuscular patients. However, laboratory research [49] demonstrates that the endotracheal tube or tracheostomy tube substantially increases resistance to airflow as narrower is the diameter of the artificial airway. Hence, higher insufflation/exsufflation pressures (e.g. up to 60–70 cmH_2O) may be necessaries to ensure adequate peak expiratory flows in the critically ill on IMV. Finally, different in-exsufflation time and inspiratory flow velocity (i.e. fast or slow) has been used in the literature. Indeed, rapid inspiratory flows with 2–3 s of inspiratory time and 3–4 s of expiratory time are currently proposed. However, in vitro and animal experimental studies objectively assessing artificial airway secretions demonstrated that slow inspiratory flows, prolonged insufflation time compared to exsufflation time (i.e. 4 and 3 s, respectively) and a gradient of pressure in favour of exsufflation pressure (i.e. +40/−70 cmH_2O) may optimise expiratory-inspiratory flow bias and promote outward clearance of mucus [50, 51]. Furthermore, recent animal data indicates that insufflation pressures of +50 cmH_2O may promote inward movement of mucus and generate a deleterious but transient increase of transpulmonary inspiratory pressure [51].

Although more studies on the best MI-E setting for the critically ill are warranted, it is suggested to modify the parameters of the device to achieve a sufficient expiratory-inspiratory flow bias.

2.5 Inspiratory Muscle Training

During invasive mechanical ventilation, diaphragm activity is partially or fully supported by the ventilator, resulting in a rapid diaphragmatic dysfunction. This critical condition, denominated ventilator-induced diaphragm dysfunction (VIDD), is detectable after 18–69 h of mechanical ventilation and affects up to 65% of all invasively ventilated patients [52]. IMV for more than 18 h is correlated with early diaphragm fibre atrophy, a decrease in cross-sectional areas of 57% of slow-twitch fibres and 53% of fast-twitch fibres [51]. Moreover, in the worst-case scenarios, diaphragmatic dysfunction can lead to a weight loss of the diaphragm, disorganisation of sarcomere's structure, increased oxidative stress and proteolysis [53, 54]. Thus, VIDD is directly related to the time spent under mechanical ventilation and the ventilatory mode. Indeed, diaphragmatic dysfunction is most evident in patients ventilated through controlled modes (i.e. continuous mandatory ventilation) than assisted-controlled modes (i.e. intermittent mandatory ventilation), whilst continuous spontaneous ventilation (e.g. pressure support ventilation) seems to minimise the structural damage [55]. Conversely, diaphragmatic oxidative stress can result from all modalities of ventilation including continuous spontaneous modes such as pressure support ventilation [53, 55]. Additionally, patients ventilated for more than 24 h may also present a decrease in diaphragmatic twitch pressure (Pditw), which is considered as the *Gold Standard* to measure involuntary diaphragm contractility. Of note, Pditw consists of a bilateral magnetic stimulation of phrenic nerves at their anterolateral neck path and 10 cmH_2O is considered the threshold for normal contractility in intubated and critically ill patients [53, 54]. Low Pditw is correlated with VIDD and often present in patients ventilated during prolonged periods with higher associated rates of weaning and extubation failure [54]. Finally, there is growing evidence of the use of Ultrasound to identify diaphragm atrophy, by its thickness or excursion changes, being, by its easy use, a promising tool to monitorise the IMT as well [56].

During the last decade, a growing body of evidence suggests inspiratory muscle training (IMT) as a potential strategy to improve the strength of inspiratory muscles and minimise their impairment during IMV. IMT consists in resistive inspiratory manoeuvres through a mechanical device comprising a unidirectional valve that hinders inspiration [18]. The therapy has been demonstrated to reverse respiratory muscle weakness and enhance the endurance of the diaphragm. Clinically this is associated with increased maximal inspiratory pressure (MIP), increased likelihood of weaning success and decreased length of stay in difficult-to-wean patients who repeatedly failed spontaneous breathing trials and/or extubation [18]. Although IMT is reported to be safe with no related adverse respiratory events and/or hemodynamic instability, the manoeuvre is not exempt of concerns since the patient-ventilator disconnection is required. Therefore, IMT is suggested for patients on IMV for ≥ 7 days, provided that described parameters for clinical stability are present (Table 2.4) [19].

Table 2.4 Parameters of clinical stability to perform inspiratory muscle training

• The patient is alert and cooperative
• Body temperature >36.5 and $\leq 38.5\ ^{\circ}$C
• PEEP ≤ 10 cmH$_2$O
• FiO$_2$ <60%
• Respiratory rate <25 bpm
• PaO$_2$ >60 mmHg and SpO$_2$ >90%
• The patient is able to trigger spontaneous breaths

Adapted from "Bisset BM, Leditschke IA, Neeman T, Boots R, Paratz J. Inspiratory muscle training to enhance recovery from mechanical ventilation: a randomised trial. Thorax 2016;71:812–819" and "Martin AD, Smith BK, Davenport PD, Harman E, Gonzalez-Rothi RJ, Baz M, et al. Inspiratory muscle strength training improves weaning outcome in failure to wean patients: a randomised trial. Crit Care 2011;15: R84"

PEEP positive en-expiratory pressure, *F$_I$O$_2$* fraction of inspired oxygen, *PaO$_2$* arterial partial pressure of oxygen, *SpO$_2$* pulse oximeter oxygen saturation, *bpm* breath per minute

IMT methods described along with the literature usually consist of 6–30 repetitions (e.g. 3 sets of 10 repetitions) with an initial resistive load up to 30–50% of the previously measured MIP, to then be increased to the highest tolerable intensity allowing consecution of most of the repetitions [19–21]. Importantly, a 1-min pause between series is allowed to reconnect the patient to mechanical ventilation and avoid the risk of oxygen desaturation. MIP should be revaluated daily to readjust the resistive load if necessary, increasing the intensity by 10% or 1–2 cmH$_2$O each new MIP. Finally, if baseline MIP is not measurable, IMT load can be titrated manually via a "trial-and-error" method, where the device is regulated at a low intensity (e.g. 9 cmH$_2$O) to then progressively increase resistance until the patient can only complete up to 6 breaths during a set of repetitions [21]. The most challenging situation associated with this approach is that the patient must be awake and participative.

Other strategies have been proposed to increase inspiratory muscle load, such as modification of trigger sensitivity or a decrease of the pressure support; however, these studies resulted in non-significant differences in any of the outcomes assessed. The proposition that the pressure delivered to the lungs during IMV is a cumulative effect of the pressure generated by the muscular system and the mechanical pressure from the ventilator appears to be theoretically and conceptually plausible, new evidence to validate this rational in clinical practice is necessary [57].

Key Take Home Messages

- Critically ill patients on invasive mechanical ventilation often present retention of airway secretions with endotracheal intubation considered as the primary mechanism.
- During invasive mechanical ventilation, the delivery of supplemental heat and moisture is highly recommended to prevent damage of the airway mucosa.
- Endotracheal suctioning is not exempt from associated complications and should be performed according to current guidelines.
- Chest physiotherapy aims to enhance mucus clearance in the critically ill, nowadays, through techniques that modulate the airflows and improve expiratory-inspiratory flow bias.
- Respiratory muscle training during invasive mechanical ventilation is feasible and may facilitate weaning in selected population of patients.

References

1. Konrad F, Schreiber T, Brecht-Kraus D, et al. Mucociliary transport in ICU patients. Chest. 1994;105:237–41.
2. Shah C, Kollef MH. Endotracheal tube intraluminal volume loss among mechanically ventilated patients. Crit Care Med. 2004;32:120–5.
3. Shapiro M, Wilson RK, Casar G, Bloom K, Teague RB. Work of breathing through different sized endotracheal tubes. Crit Care Med. 1986;14:1028–31.

4. Sackner MA, Hirsch J, Epstein S. Effect of cuffed endotracheal tubes on tracheal mucous velocity. Chest. 1975;68:774–7.
5. Gal TJ. Effects of endotracheal intubation on normal cough performance. Anesthesiology. 1980;52:324–9.
6. Kilgour E, Rankin N, Ryan S, Pack R. Mucociliary function deteriorates in the clinical range of inspired air temperature and humidity. Intensive Care Med. 2004;30(7):1491–4.
7. Cole AM, Dewan P, Ganz T. Innate antimicrobial activity of nasal secretions. Infect Immun. 1999;67:3267–75.
8. Dullenkopf A, Gerber A, Weiss M. Fluid leakage past tracheal tube cuffs: evaluation of the new microcuff endotracheal tube. Intensive Care Med. 2003;29:1849–53.
9. Torres A, Serra-Batlles J, Ros E, Piera C, de la Puig BJ, Cobos A, et al. Pulmonary aspiration of gastric contents in patients receiving mechanical ventilation: the effect of body position. Ann Intern Med. 1992;116:540–3.
10. Drakulovic MB, Torres A, Bauer TT, Nicolas JM, Nogue S, Ferrer M. Supine body position as a risk factor for nosocomial pneumonia in mechanically ventilated patients: a randomised trial. Lancet. 1999;354:1851–8.
11. American Thoracic Society, Infectious Diseases Society of America. Guidelines for the management of adults with hospital-acquired, ventilator-associated, and healthcare-associated pneumonia. Am J Respir Crit Care Med. 2005;171:388–416.
12. Li Bassi G, Zanella A, Cressoni M, Stylianou M, Kolobow T. Following tracheal intubation, mucus flow is reversed in the semirecumbent position: possible role in the pathogenesis of ventilator-associated pneumonia. Crit Care Med. 2008;36:518–25.
13. Latronico N, Bolton CF. Critical illness polyneuropathy and myopathy: a major cause of muscle weakness and paralysis. Lancet Neurol. 2011;10:931–41.
14. Jolley SE, Bunnell AE, Hough CL. ICU-acquired weakness. Chest. 2016;150:1129–40.
15. De Jonghe B, Bastuji-Garin S, Durand MC, Malissin I, Rodrigues P, Cerf C, et al. Respiratory weakness is associated with limb weakness and delayed weaning in critical illness. Crit Care Med. 2007;35:2007–15.
16. Supinski GS, Morris PE, Dhar S, Callahan LA. Diaphragm dysfunction in critical illness. Chest. 2018;153:1040–51.
17. Hodgson CL, Tipping CJ. Physiotherapy management of intensive care unit-acquired weakness. J Physiother. 2017;63:4–10.
18. Elkins M, Dentice R. Inspiratory muscle training facilitates weaning from mechanical ventilation among patients in the intensive care unit: a systematic review. J Physiother. 2015;61:125–34.
19. Marques Tonella R, Roceto Ratti LDS, Delazari LEB, Junior CF, Da Silva PL, Herran ARDS, et al. Inspiratory muscle training in the intensive care unit: a new perspective. J Clin Med Res. 2017;9:929–34.
20. Bisset BM, Leditschke IA, Neeman T, Boots R, Paratz J. Inspiratory muscle training to enhance recovery from mechanical ventilation: a randomised trial. Thorax. 2016;71:812–9.
21. Martin AD, Smith BK, Davenport PD, Harman E, Gonzalez-Rothi RJ, Baz M, et al. Inspiratory muscle strength training improves weaning outcome in failure to wean patients: a randomized trial. Crit Care. 2011;15:R84.
22. Blakeman TC, Scott JB, Yoder MA, Capellari E, Strickland SL. AARC clinical practice guidelines: artificial airway suctioning. Respir Care. 2022;67(2):258–71.
23. Guglielminotti J, Alzieu M, Maury E, Guidet B, Offenstadt G. Bedside detection of retained tracheobronchial secretions in patients receiving mechanical ventilation: is it time for tracheal suctioning? Chest. 2000;118:1095–9.
24. Caruso P, Denari S, Ruiz SA, Demarzo SE, Deheinzelin D. Saline instillation before tracheal suctioning decreases the incidence of ventilator-associated pneumonia. Crit Care Med. 2009;37:32–8.
25. Ramírez-Torres CA, Rivera-Sanz F, Sufrate-Sorzano T, Pedraz-Marcos A, Santolalla-Arnedo I. Closed endotracheal suction systems for COVID-19: rapid review. Interact J Med Res. 2023;12:e42549.

26. Frost SA, Azeem A, Alexandrou E, Tam V, Murphy JK, Hunt L, et al. Subglottic secretion drainage for preventing ventilator associated pneumonia: a meta-analysis. Aust Crit Care. 2013;26:180–8.

27. Tomaszek L, Pawlik J, Mazurek H, Mędrzycka-Dąbrowska W. Automatic continuous control of cuff pressure and subglottic secretion suction used together to prevent pneumonia in ventilated patients—a retrospective and prospective cohort study. J Clin Med. 2021;10(21):4952. https://doi.org/10.3390/jcm10214952.

28. AARC, Restrepo RD, Walsh BK. Humidification during invasive and noninvasive mechanical ventilation. Respir Care. 2012;57:782–8.

29. Kelly M, Gillies D, Todd DA, Lockwood C. Heated humidification versus heat and moisture exchangers for ventilated adults and children. Cochrane Database Syst Rev. 2010;(4):CD004711.

30. Branson RD. Secretion management in the mechanically ventilated patient. Respir Care. 2007;52:1328–42.

31. Stiller K. Physiotherapy in intensive care: towards an evidence-based practice. Chest. 2000;118:1801–13.

32. Stiller K. Physiotherapy in intensive care: an updated systematic review. Chest. 2013;144:825–47.

33. Benjamin RG, Chapman GA, Kim CS, Sackner MA. Removal of bronchial secretions by two-phase gas-liquid transport. Chest. 1989;95:658–63.

34. Kim CS, Rodriguez CR, Eldridge MA, Sackner MA. Criteria for mucus transport in the airways by two-phase gas-liquid flow mechanism. J Appl Physiol. 1986;60:901–7.

35. Kim CS, Greene MA, Sankaran S, Sackner MA. Mucus transport in the airways by two-phase gas-liquid flow mechanism: continuous flow model. J Appl Physiol. 1986;60:908–17.

36. Kim CS, Iglesias AJ, Sackner MA. Mucus clearance by two-phase gas-liquid flow mechanism: asymmetric periodic flow model. J Appl Physiol. 1987;62:959–71.

37. Denehy L. The use of manual hyperinflation in airway clearance. Eur Respir J. 1999;14:958–65.

38. Valer BB, Bonczynski GS, Scheffer KD, Ibrahim Forgiarini SG, Eibel B, Lisboa Cordeiro AL, Friedman G, Forgiarini Júnior LA. Ventilator versus manual hyperinflation in adults receiving mechanical ventilation: a systematic review. Physiother Res Int. 2022;27(2):e1936.

39. Martinez BP, Lobo LL, de Queiroz RS, Saquetto MB, Júnior LAF, Correia HF, Silva CMSE, Alves IGN, Neto MG. Effects of ventilator hyperinflation on pulmonary function and secretion clearance in adults receiving mechanical ventilation: a systematic review with meta-analysis. Heart Lung. 2022;56:8–23.

40. Volpe MS, Guimarães FS, Morais CC. Airway clearance techniques for mechanically ventilated patients: insights for optimization. Respir Care. 2020;65(8):1174–88.

41. Borges LF, Saraiva MS, Saraiva MAS, Macagnan FE, Kessler A. Expiratory rib cage compression in mechanically ventilated adults: systematic review with meta-analysis. Rev Bras Ter Intensiva. 2017;29:96–104.

42. Guimarães FS, Lopes AJ, Constantino SS, Lima JC, Canuto P, de Menezes SL. Expiratory rib cage compression in mechanically ventilated subjects: a randomized crossover trial [corrected]. Respir Care. 2014;59:678–85.

43. Ouchi A, Sakuramoto H, Unoki T, Yoshino Y, Hosino H, Koyama Y, Enomoto Y, Shimojo N, Mizutani T, Inoue Y. Effects of manual rib cage compressions on mucus clearance in mechanically ventilated pigs. Respir Care. 2020;65(8):1135–40.

44. Martí JD, Bassi GL, Rigol M, Saucedo L, Ranzani OT, Esperatti M, et al. Effects of manual rib cage compressions on expiratory flow and mucus clearance during mechanical ventilation. Crit Care Med. 2013;41:850–6.

45. Homnick DN. Mechanical insufflation-exsufflation for airway mucus clearance. Respir Care. 2007;52:1296–305.

46. Martínez-Alejos R, Martí JD, Li Bassi G, Gonzalez-Anton D, Pilar-Diaz X, Reginault T, Wibart P, Ntoumenopoulos G, Tronstad O, Gabarrus A, Quinart A, Torres A. Effects of mechanical insufflation-exsufflation on sputum volume in mechanically ventilated critically ill subjects. Respir Care. 2021;66(9):1371–9. https://doi.org/10.4187/respcare.08641.

47. Ferreira de Camillis ML, Savi A, Goulart Rosa R, Figueiredo M, Wickert R, Borges LGA, et al. Effects of mechanical insufflation-exsufflation on airway mucus clearance among mechanically ventilated ICU subjects. Respir Care. 2018;63:1471–7.
48. Coutinho WM, Vieira PJC, Kutchak FM, Dias AS, Rieder MM, Forgiarini LA Jr. Comparison of mechanical insufflation-exsufflation and endotracheal suctioning in mechanically ventilated patients: effects on respiratory mechanics, hemodynamics, and volume of secretions. Indian J Crit Care Med. 2018;22:485–90.
49. Guerin C, Bourdin G, Leray V, Delannoy B, Bayle F, Germain M, Richard JC. Performance of the cough assist insufflation-exsufflation device in the presence of an endotracheal tube or tracheostomy tube: a bench study. Respir Care. 2011;56:1108–14.
50. Volpe MS, Naves JM, Ribeiro GG, Ruas G, Amato MBP. Airway clearance with an optimized mechanical insufflation-exsufflation maneuver. Respir Care. 2018;63:1214–22.
51. Martí JD, Martínez-Alejos R, Pilar-Diaz X, Yang H, Pagliara F, Battaglini D, Meli A, Yang M, Bobi J, Rigol M, Tronstad O, Volpe MS, Passos Amato MB, Bassi GL, Torres A. Effects of mechanical insufflation-exsufflation with different pressure settings on respiratory mucus displacement during invasive ventilation. Respir Care. 2022;67(12):1508–16.
52. Levine S, Nguyen T, Taylor N, Friscia M, Budak MT, Rothenberg P, et al. Rapid disuse atrophy of diaphragm fibers in mechanically ventilated humans. N Engl J Med. 2007;358:1327–35.
53. Tobin MJ, Laghi F, Jubran A. Narrative review: ventilator-induced respiratory muscle weakness. Ann Intern Med. 2010;153:240–5.
54. Jaber S, Petrof BJ, Jung B, Chanques G, Berthet J, Rabel C, et al. Rapidly progressive diaphragmatic weakness and injury during mechanical ventilation in humans. Am J Respir Crit Care Med. 2011;183:364–71.
55. Marin-Corral J, Dot I, Boguña M, Cecchini L, Zapatero A, Gracia MP, et al. Structural differences in the diaphragm of patients following controlled vs assisted and spontaneous mechanical ventilation. Intensive Care Med. 2019;45:488–500.
56. Truong D, Abo S, Whish-Wilson GA, D'Souza AN, Beach LJ, Mathur S, Mayer KP, Ntoumenopoulos G, Baldwin C, El-Ansary D, Paris MT, Mourtzakis M, Morris PE, Pastva AM, Granger CL, Parry SM, Sarwal A. Methodological and clinimetric evaluation of inspiratory respiratory muscle ultrasound in the critical care setting: a systematic review and meta-analysis. Crit Care Med. 2023;51(2):e24–36.
57. Caruso P, Denari SD, Ruiz SA, Bernal KG, Manfrin GM, Friedrich C, Deheinzelin D. Inspiratory muscle training is ineffective in mechanically ventilated critically ill patients. Clinics (Sao Paulo). 2005;60(6):479–84.

Silvia Calviño-Günther and Yann Vallod

3.1 Introduction: Patient Care in a Critical Environment

Intensive care is a highly complex and technological environment, with increasing demands placed on clinical staff to provide optimal organ support and lifesaving treatment. Consequently, some of the perceived lower-valued tasks (e.g. bathing, bed care, urinary catheter care) may not be considered as a nursing priority, often delegated to healthcare assistants. This has led to a culture where the importance of direct patient care may no longer be emphasised, and healthcare workers risk detaching themselves from the fundamental needs of patients to invest in more technical aspects [1]. However, it is precisely this direct care that allows care providers to proceed to a thorough patient assessment, and all these 'less valued' tasks which have a definite impact in detecting any threat to the patients' defences, a lack of adaptation to the environment, or any other kind of insult, from skin integrity to pain, agitation or anxiety [2].

The model of medical and nursing care has switched from being focused initially only on the diagnosis and treatment of acute illness, to the improvement of outcomes, prevention of iatrogenic complications, and hospital-acquired conditions, and to help increase patient comfort and well-being. Reviews of hospital data analyzing all preventable errors identify up to 63% related to clinical issues that are 'nursing sensitive' and can be measured [3–5]; in this category, we could include many hospital-acquired conditions (HAC) including:

- Skin injuries.
- Post-operative respiratory complications.
- Falls.
- Use of restraints.
- Hospital-acquired infections.

S. Calviño-Günther (✉) · Y. Vallod
Medical Intensive Care Unit, University Hospital of Grenoble-Alpes, Grenoble, France

© The Author(s), under exclusive license to Springer Nature Switzerland AG 2024
C. Boulanger, D. McWilliams (eds.), *Passport to Successful Outcomes for Patients Admitted to ICU*, https://doi.org/10.1007/978-3-031-53019-7_3

Specifically when considering hospital-acquired infections (HAI), the focus will be on the so-called Big Four (see Box 3.1).

Box 3.1 The 'Big Four' of Hospital-Acquired Infections
- Catheter-associated urinary tract infections (CAUTI).
- Central-line associated blood-stream infections (CLABSI).
- Ventilator-associated pneumonia (VAP).
- Surgical site infections (SSI).

However, despite the fact that the reduction of these events has a major impact on improving outcomes, it would be very reductive to resume patients' care only to prevent avoidable errors. Even if one of the main objectives is to give back its place and its value to these essential nursing tasks which are the foundation of clinical, bedside nursing practice, global patient care has a much higher scope. In particular, in critical settings, the aim of patient care is to create an atmosphere of comfort, physical and mental ease, reduce stressors, and restore the patients' place and dignity in the middle of a setting where technology and innovation seem to reign without sharing [6, 7].

The aim of this chapter is to review evidence-based, fundamental nursing interventions in critical care to maintain the clinical condition and support health recovery. Under the global term of 'patient care', the aim is to provide an atmosphere of comfort, and physical and mental ease, enabling interventions such as hygiene, infection prevention, pain and anxiety control, while respecting patient's values [6]. The maintenance of these elements through reflexive care is a fundamental responsibility of caregivers and will have a significant impact on clinical outcomes, patient and family satisfaction, quality of care and ultimately successful discharge.

Our objective is also to include patient care, even in a critical setting, in a broader perspective. This might start with the WHO definition for quality care, as mentioned before [8]; or we try to go further, for instance, defining patient care in the scope of Picker's 'Eight Principles of quality patient-centered care' [9] (See Fig. 3.1). This clinical evaluation will not assess only vital constants, but also coordinates and organises care within the whole structure; it has to observe, listen and take into account patient's reactions, even the slightest alteration in their state, needs, comfort and well-being. This comprehensive, respectful, evidence-based and patient-centred approach by the care team will assure a positive impact on outcomes.

As the issue is extremely wide, specific items like infection control, environmental impact or communication will be addressed in separate chapters. This chapter will specifically focus on two fundamental aspects of basic care: interventional patient hygiene, and interventions to prevent and/or reduce stressors and emotional insults due to pain and agitation.

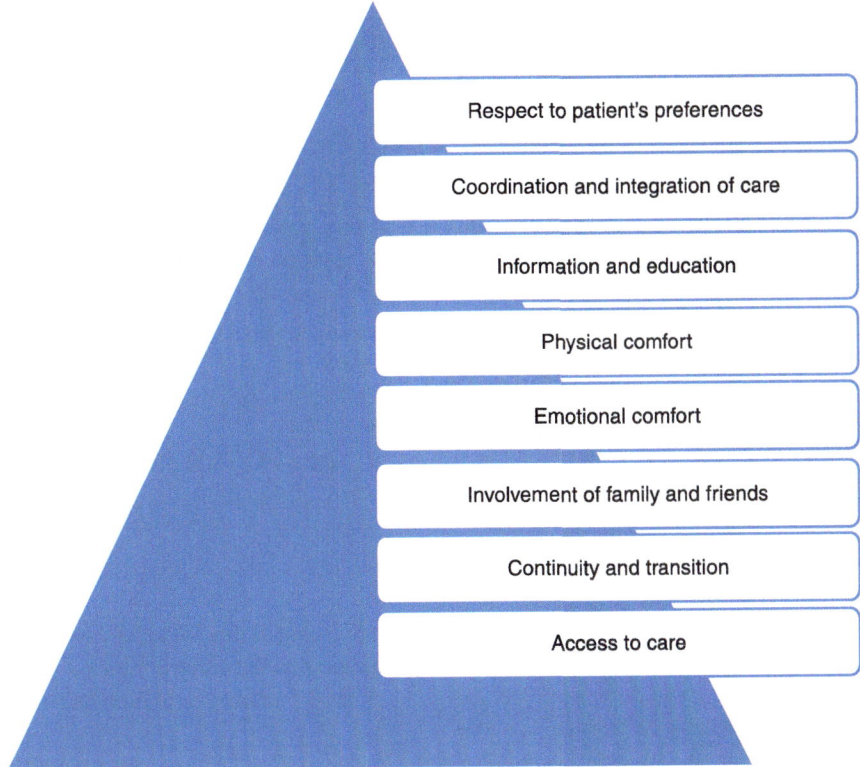

Fig. 3.1   Picker's eight principles of quality of patient centred-care

3.2   'Interventional Patient Hygiene'

The management of technical and sophisticated equipment and an increasing number of administrative tasks have a large impact on the workload of care providers [10]. However as many of these nursing interventions have a definite impact on the occurrence (or even better, prevention) of HAC and HAI, and also because in some countries insurances companies refuse to reimburse costs related to preventable adverse events, basic patient care has recently taken a new lease, with a trend that could be actually be called 'back to the basics' [2, 3, 11].

The works of Vollman et al. [2] can be considered as the core of this approach, defining and developing the Interventional Patient Hygiene (IPH) model (see Fig. 3.2). This model provided a nursing action plan for the critical care environment, 'directly oriented on fortifying patients' host defenses through the use of evidence-based care'. Vollman's work stressed the importance of fundamental care interventions such as hygiene, always building on evidence-based knowledge as the basis for obtaining the highest levels of safety and quality. The initial model was

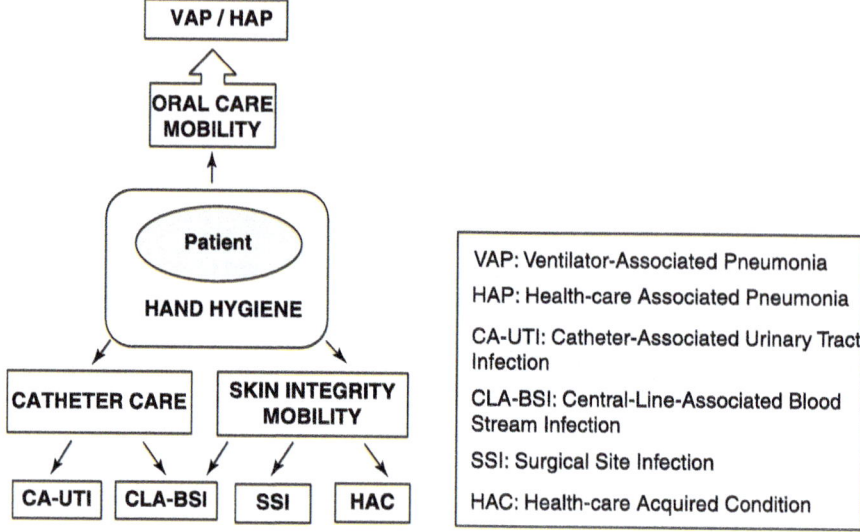

Fig. 3.2 Based on the Interventional Patient Hygiene Model: a conceptual framework [3]

focused on two real-life, evidence-based hygiene bundles that included oral care, bathing, incontinence management and mobility, and demonstrated a real impact on preventing the development of ventilator-associated pneumonia (VAP), pressure ulcers and perineal dermatitis.

The original model was progressively broadened [3, 12] to include care providers hand hygiene (an essential practice to reduce the bioburden of both the patient and the care provider) and skin antisepsis/catheter care, two extremely sensitive nursing interventions that have a direct impact on health-care acquired infections (HAIs).

Interventional patient hygiene (IPH) might be regarded as a routine task; however they demand careful assessment of patient's needs, the aims, risks, and benefits of every intervention. The concept of IPH emphasises basic nursing functions are not only tasks, but important evidence-based interventions which contribute to improve patient outcomes, integrating science and practice. These interventions, placed in the context of a comprehensive program for reducing error, may help prioritise a list of care activities for critical care nurses. It demands real scientific analysis of the impact of nursing interventions on everyday outcomes, a deep reflection on the priorities of nursing care in ICU, and the awareness of the importance of basic nursing care. Some of the interventions such as hand hygiene, catheter care and mobility will be extensively explored in further chapters; in this chapter, for the physical aspects of patient care, there will be a focus on bathing and skin integrity, and oral care.

3.3 Bathing and Skin Integrity

Skin preservation, (including bathing, bed-care, basic mobilisation, and therapeutic touch), is one of the most frequent and holistic nursing interventions in Intensive Care. The aims are multiple and simultaneous: ensuring personal hygiene, formal skin wound and dressings assessment, preventing hospital-acquired conditions, reducing pyrexia, stimulating circulation and, of course, promoting comfort, relaxation, and well-being for the patient. It is considered *a privileged moment in that it also represents a moment of intimacy and communication between the patient and the caregivers.* It is, therefore, surprising to observe that for such an important and frequent procedure, there are so few evidence-based recommendations to determine timing, duration, cleansing agents, or even frequency, and a paucity of literature about the impact of this practice on patients, either in the positive or negative.

If a patient-centred pattern is followed, patients should receive the level of assistance that they require to meet their individual personal hygiene needs. This in itself may be a delicate issue, needs vary between individuals and cultures, creating the potential for conflict between patients' needs and the unit procedures and habits. It is worth noting that, as most of the ICU patients are sedated, bed bath timing is mostly chosen with regard to the units' needs and habits, and patients or their surrogates are rarely consulted about their particular needs or preferences [13]. Therefore, it is not unusual that bathing procedures take place during the night duty, between 2 and 6 a.m. due to workload, organisational factors or personnel restrictions [14], precisely at a moment when REM sleep periods, the more resting, should take place. Sleep deprivation is one of the most common insults in intensive care, and interventions like bathing (as well as other procedures, like suctioning, electrograph recording, catheter care) participate intensively in this fragmentation [15, 16]. Critical patients experience an overexposure to light, the most powerful reference for the circadian time system, but many other non-photic cues, like mealtime, physical activity and social interactions are disrupted in ICU, that contribute to desynchronisation of the biological clock.

There is still a debate whether even without these night procedures, critically ill patient's sleep could improve, as already medication, mechanical ventilation and, of course, their instable condition and the ICU environment have a large part in the responsibility of sleep disturbances [15, 16]. Nonetheless, current recommendations propose to re-establish circadian rhythms for patients by organising most of these invasive procedures during daytime and there is a growing body of literature testing sleeping promotion protocols, reducing the number of nursing procedures at particular moments of the night [17–20].

Bathing in the stressful setting of the ICU, and particularly if interrupting a moment of rest, can be a source of anxiety and fear; caregivers should take this into account whenever possible for planning their tasks, to propose a safe and comfortable moment of care. Although the provision of a daily bath is a usual practice in intensive care, patients' haemodynamic stability, continence or the prioritisation of other interventions can alter this periodicity. Unanswered is whether daily bathing with the traditional basin, soap and tap water procedure can be considered as best practice. Nurses still learn to bed-bath patients routinely with a basin; however, studies in the United Kingdom, the United States and Canada have demonstrated sound evidence that tap water is *'a major offender in the development of waterborne pathogen infections in acute care hospitals'* [21] and others also point out at most bath basins at hospital, as a possible reservoir of pathogens that might play a role in spreading HAI in critically ill patients [22]. There is a consensus in avoiding alkaline soaps, as they alter the natural skin composition. The use of disposable wash-clothes has shown to reduce skin contamination, but no significant reduction of HAI [23], and there have been some large and promising trials, *both in medical and in surgical settings,* proposing the use of chlorhexidine (CHG) impregnated wash cloths to reduce multi-resistant pathogen transmission [24, 25]. However the latest Cochrane Systematic review on the subject [26] concluded the evidence of the efficacy of CHG on HAI, mortality, or any other outcome, or even if there are more skin-related adverse events, remains very low, as most studies were downgraded for performance bias, inconsistency, imprecision or study limitations. As for other studies, there is still an absence of sufficient not enough evidence on a particular cleansing agent recommended for bed-bathing critically ill patients.

There is a strong consensus on the use of topical moisturizers and emollients after bathing, in particular in patients with dry or flaky skin, to prevent pressure ulcers. Despite this, the literature suggests that these are still insufficiently used in critical settings. It is recommended moisturizers and emollients should be used after bathing, but also at bed-care moments, during positioning or turning, combined with a slight massage to induce relaxation and give a moment of comfort.

Last but not least, caring for a patient in a critical care setting includes the need to help them to get the most natural and comfortable position, and reposition them regularly in particular when sedated or under blocking agents. This careful, therapeutic repositioning allows the caregiver to assess skin integrity, reduce pressure injuries and keep some joint flexibility. Although no specific guidelines are written, it is currently accepted that repositioning sedated patients should take place every 2–4 h. Positioning is equally important, respecting the body axel, avoiding hyperextension of the neck with an appropriate pillow, placing the patient (unless a medical contraindication) in a semi-recumbent position that will help ventilatory movements, while respecting the natural position of shoulders, hips, knees, ankles, and leaving some movement possible.

3.4 Oral Care

In normal conditions, the oral system (i.e. mouth/throat) has a cleansing process of its own, where salivation, chewing and swallowing have an important role. This way, deposits in the mouth are reduced, and part of these elements is pre-digested through the enzymes contained in saliva, stimulated by chewing. Ventilated and sedated critically ill patients are unable to fulfil this role. The mouth, open and often congested by intubation or feeding tubes, cannot ensure this physiological process, leading to an accumulation of bacteria within the oral cavity, often accompanied by microlesions due to the presence of foreign devices and mucosa dryness.

The care providers' role is, therefore, to support optimal regulation, bringing the oral cavity to an apparent normality. This includes performing suction as required in case of over-salivation; mouthwash and rinses for teeth, tongue, palate, and gums for reducing mouth dryness, also the prevention of pressure ulcers or damaged skin and mucosa through close monitoring of the various tubes.

Besides the positive impact from a physiological perspective, mouth care should be noted as being a psychologically positive intervention in terms of comfort and well-being. In this respect, paediatric and palliative care teams have shown the lead with the development of specific protocols and constant research when caring for patients in a state of dependence and extreme weakness. Frequent oral evaluation and the use of individualised protocols for oral care are essential to preserve oral hygiene and comfort, and reduce mouth dryness. Studies in this area however have important limitations, with wide variability in measures of material, cleansing agents used or frequency of interventions. The small cohorts also limit the wider generalisation of results obtained. Recent research in intensive care has focused on the impact of oral care in the reduction of ventilator-associated pneumonia (VAP) with promising results [2], although other research on this topic has explored the different symptoms evidenced by patients such as mouth dryness and thirst, and the interventions that could alleviate them [27]. Evidence supports the use of swabs or soft-bristled toothbrushes, or even of ice chips, depending on the needs of the patient, and rinsing the oral cavity carefully at a frequency that varies from 2- to 12-h intervals, although it seems that 2- and 4-h intervals improve oral hygiene, and increase in this interval might lose most of the benefits.

In recent years, research has tried to reduce ventilator-associated pneumonia through the implementation of prevention bundles, often including oral hygiene interventions. There is an innovative research in this field, still in its beginnings, testing photodynamic therapy, NO-based therapy, anti-virulence therapy and other antimicrobial strategies. Nevertheless, the most studied procedure is still the use of chlorhexidine rinses, as a simple, low-cost approach to VAP prophylaxis. Lately, chlorhexidine has also been used in oncology and immunocompromised patients, and actually up to 70% of intensive care units across Europe and North America perform daily oral care with chlorhexidine. Studies supporting these interventions have still strong limitations (little samples, bias related to group analysis or lack of agreement in the VAP definition), so generalisation of those findings is often difficult, and there is no strong supporting evidence for the use of any particular cleansing agent. Subsequently, there exist no recommendation for their use. CHORAL, a recent study on de-adoption of chlorhexidine rinse, failed also to find a difference in mortality or ventilator-associated conditions either in the chlorhexidine group or in the oral care bundle group [28]. Further research on the subject is strongly needed, to propose robust and sound guidelines on this fundamental intervention [29].

3.5   Eye Care

'The eyes are the mirror of the soul and reflect everything that seems to be hidden; and like a mirror, they also reflect the person looking into them' (Paolo Coelho, *Manuscript Found in Accra*). Many philosophers and writers brilliantly described our particular relationship to this organ. Sight is the most developed sensory organ, and up to 80% of all impressions arrive at our brain through the eyes; when one of the other senses is impaired, the eyes will take over to protect us from danger. Not

only the function is important, but the eyes have a special place in our lives. Nevertheless, they are not a vital organ and, during an acute episode, their care can be moved to the background, allowing the occurrence of painful and sometimes serious complications which can impact negatively in the post ICU phase.

Eyes have also their own physiological mechanisms to protect them from environmental damage; this natural defense includes tear formation, eye blinking and eye closure [30]. Tears play an essential role, as they maintain a moist environment that prevents drying of the thin conjunctival membrane; they also remove dust particles, deliver immune cells and antibodies and lubricate the eyelids. Blinking and eyelids closure participate in the mechanical defense against trauma, while distributing tears and sweeping away debris. Eye closure is actually an active process, and the inability to perform efficient closure, known as lagophthalmos, is a frequent disorder in mechanically ventilated patients, mostly due to the use of sedative agents that inhibit natural defenses [30, 31]. Lagophthalmos, as well as other ICU conditions like conjunctival oedema, prone positioning or mechanical positive pressure ventilation, are important precipitating risk factors leading to ocular surface disease (OSD).

The incidence of ocular surface disease ranges from 23% up to 60% of critically ill patients and can affect any structure of the eye, including the sclera and the conjunctival epithelium [30]. The most common disorders include superficial corneal abrasion, exposure keratopathy and chemosis or conjunctival swelling; more serious but less often aggressions are microbial conjunctivitis and keratitis, corneal lacerations, cataracts, pressure effects, and visual loss.

Nursing procedures should, therefore, include a careful assessment of the eyes, and the introduction of specific care procedures will depend on the patients' condition and the ability to maintain the eyes' physiological defense. An example of outline eye care procedure for patients mechanically ventilated is given in Table 3.1. They might need both mechanical methods to close the eyelids and protect the cornea when the closure is impaired, and/or 4 to 2 hourly eye care to clean the eye surface and moist them with topical moisturizers and lubricants. There are a wide variety of products to prevent corneal dryness and maintain the protective moisture

Table 3.1 Eye care procedure for mechanically ventilated patients with a GCS <10

Grade	Action
0: Eyes Defence ON	Check whether eyelids close efficiently at least every 4 h
1: Eyes Defence PARTIALLY ON	Eyes need systematic care every 2–4 h: • Clean the eyes surface with sterile gauze moistened with saline solution • Check corneal clarity • Instill ointment/lubricant
2: Eyes Defence OFF	Eyes need artificial lubricating and lids taping • Clean the surface of eyes with sterile gauze moistened with saline solution • Check corneal clarity • Instill ointment/lubricant • Close lids artificially

film, as methylcellulose drops or ointment, polyacrylamide gel, hypromellose drops (also known as artificial tears), paraffin gauze dressings, or even lubricating prophylactic antibiotics. In general, long-acting agents should be preferred for maximum benefits, while eyelids closure with tape should be used only as the last resort. Among the various eye care measures tested essentially to prevent keratopathy, the most effective seems to be the application of polyethylene covers [32].

Other innovative procedures include moisture chambers, which have been used and found effective when compared with standard measures. Once placed on the eye, these chambers act as a polyethylene occlusive film that protects the eye and keeps moisture in. Early results are promising, including a recent meta-analysis, but further validation is still required [33].

3.6   Pain Assessment and Nursing Care

The pain was defined in 1978 by the International Association for the Study of Painas 'an *unpleasant sensory and emotional experience related to, or described in terms of, actual or potential tissue damage*' [34]. In accordance with its impact on patients' quality of life and outcomes, the American Pain Society imposed the concept of pain as the fifth vital sign in the mid-1990s, as one of the most important indicators of the body's life-sustaining functions [35]. From 30% to 50% of patients experience pain at rest, while the percentage increases during nursing procedures [36, 37]. In addition to the unpleasant experience for the patient, non-treated pain has large consequences on different functions and symptoms: increased endogenous catecholamine activity, oxygen consumption, hyper-metabolism, immune suppression, sleep deprivation, and delirium and agitation exacerbation [37]. Significant pain also leaves a long-term imprint, as it can lead to chronic pain and its association with a higher incidence of post-traumatic stress disorder has been found in numerous studies [38–42].

Two conditions related to the ICU setting, prolonged immobility and an anxiety-provoking environment, also lead to an increased frequency and severity of perceived pain sensation. ICU patients experience neuroplastic hyperalgesia and allodynia more commonly than non-critically ill patients, contributing to the high incidence of chronic pain in ICU survivors [42].

3.6.1   Assessment

It is commonly accepted that pain assessment should be given the higher priority and all scientific societies have proposed guidelines and algorithms to increase clinical decision making [43]. The gold standard in pain assessment remains patient self-reporting; therefore, pain evaluation is an everyday challenge in ICU. Vital signs alone are poor indicators of pain, although acute changes should prompt evaluation with a validated pain assessment tool. Other physiologic measures of pain are being explored and seem promising techniques for further research, like pupillometry [44] and changes in Bispectral Index or processed EEG signals, but current research shows that best-validated tools for patients unable to self-report pain are the Behavioral Pain Scale (BPS) and the Critical Care Pain Observation Tool (CPOT) [45]. International guidelines and bundles recommend assessing pain with behavioral parameters whenever critically ill patients are unable to report their pain level [46, 47]. The BPS consists of three domains: 'facial expression', 'upper limb movement' and 'mechanical ventilator compliance'. The CPOT takes into account four behavioral categories: 'facial expression', 'body movements', 'muscle tension' and 'mechanical ventilator compliance'. These tools take into account both patient's perception and expression of pain; they are easy to implement in any intensive care setting, and have shown good validity and reliability in international studies [48–50].

3.6.2 Management

Critical care nurses need to not only be aware of research-based pain management practices, but also lead the way in implementation and continuous evaluation [51]. Adapted treatment should follow pain assessment, most of the time with the help of validated sedation and analgesia protocols, or in Pain–Agitation–Delirium (PAD) bundles [46, 47]. Pain can be divided into four categories: continuous ICU treatment-related pain/ discomfort, acute illness-related pain, intermittent procedural pain, and pre-existing chronic pain present before ICU admission. A careful evaluation will enable caregivers to manage appropriately each category. Basically, any procedure performed in the ICU may be a potential source of pain; nevertheless, recent surveys have found that care teams often underestimate the pain associated with daily care procedures and there is a significant discrepancy between the recommendations and observed practice [36, 43, 49].

  In intensive care settings, pain medications should be routinely administered in the presence of significant pain (i.e. NRS >4, BPS >5, or CPOT >3), but also be routinely administered prior to performing painful invasive procedures. Opioids are often first-line drugs, sometimes with the adjunction of Gabapentin or Carbamazepine, and non-opioid analgesic added to reduce opioid requirements and reduce opioid-related side effects [36, 37]. In some cases, systemic opioids are not enough to relieve pain in adult ICU patients, and caregivers are prompted to use other target-oriented techniques. Current PAD guidelines limit for the moment the use of regional analgesia in surgical ICU patients or with traumatic injuries, through epidural analgesia and regional techniques have proven to be efficient for aging patients with hard breathing induced by the pain associated with multiple rib fractures [52]. Epidural analgesia has nevertheless some limitations in intensive care settings, the increased risk of infection of the epidural space, for instance, and are therefore difficult to implement [53]. Peripheral nerve block techniques could also be useful for surgical ICU patients, but are contraindicated in several pathologies and compel patients to remain on specific positions [54].

  Non-pharmacological interventions proposed by critical care teams, in combination with the above-mentioned medications, may also be effective, especially in procedural pain relief [55], addressing the more psychological and emotional aspects of pain and comfort. Alternative interventions, like massage, healing touch, music therapy and even facilitating family presence, can help to reduce the perception of pain, although they cannot be considered as first-line pain treatment. 'Healing Touch' or 'Therapeutic Touch', often related to Eastern healing perceptions, is an alternative therapy based on spiritual beliefs about the vitalizing energy that flows within and around living beings; it is administered by a nurse as a non-touch intervention composed of five phases: assessment, clearisng, repatterning/treatment, balancing and, finally, a reassessment of the individual's energy fields [56, 57]. Music therapy has proven to reduce the requirements of opioids and reduce the sensation of pain [58, 59], but as for all other complementary therapies, further research is still needed as the impact and relevance in clinical practice remains unclear. These therapies cannot be considered as first-line treatment in ICU, but offer the potential benefits of low cost, ease of provision and safety, and put the relationship with the patient in the centre of care. At a different level, innovative technological approaches, as virtual reality or even electronic relaxation therapies, open new perspectives to reduce pain and stressful symptoms in ICU while reducing medication; but for the moment they have not been validated by large-scale studies and their cost remains very high [60–62].

3.7   Conclusion

Critically ill patients have many specific needs for physical, psychospiritual, socio-cultural and environmental comfort, identifying these is part of the fundamental role of critical care nursing. Nurses require the knowledge necessary to be able to find the balance between the priorities inherent to the patient's illness severity and needs of life-saving procedures, and the skill to implement them with respect to patient's needs and perspectives.

IPH models are proof that evidence-based, reflexive patient care can help staff integrate best practices while balancing the challenging priorities inherent in critical care. Beyond the patient hygicnc modcls, the asscssment of all physical, cmotional, psychospiritual and environmental stressors should also be included, as it is the case for pain. It has become urgent for caregivers to resume all these care tasks, evaluate the impact on patient outcomes and integrate them as indicators of quality of care. It is not a coincidence that during patient care professionals have the opportunity to communicate with patients, assess all these elements, identify potential threats and prevent complications. There is an urgent need, however, for robust research to determine evidence-based guidelines on all these interventions that may have a sound and definite impact on a successful outcome from ICU.

Key Take Home Messages

- Despite the highly technological environment of intensive care units, basic bedside, patient-centred care remains the cornerstone of the relationship between the patient and the critical care teams,

- Regular and careful assessment of the patient's condition: skin, eyes, mouth but also the whole-body expression of discomfort and pain, prevents complications and improves outcomes.
- Delivering all these aspects of care in a personalised and compassionate manner assist the patient in feeling both cared for and an individual.
- Research is still needed to prove the impact of these various interventions in patient outcomes.

References

1. Visintini E, Inzerillo M, Savaris M, Paravan G, Serafini M, Palese A. Factors triggering the progressive detachment of nurses toward the fundamental needs of patients: findings from a qualitative study. Intern Emerg Med. 2023;18(5):1349–57.
2. Vollman K, Garcia R, Miller L. Interventional patient hygiene: proactive (hygiene) strategies to improve patients' outcomes. Education 2003;2004.
3. Vollman KM. Interventional patient hygiene: discussion of the issues and a proposed model for implementation of the nursing care basics. Intensive Crit Care Nurs. 2013;29(5):250–5.
4. Burns SM, Day T. A return to the basics: "Interventional Patient Hygiene" (a call for papers). Intensive Crit Care Nurs. 2012;28(4):193–6.
5. Burns SM, Day T. A return to the basics: 'Interventional Patient Hygiene'. Intensive Crit Care Nurs. 2013 Oct;29(5):247–9.
6. Carvajal Carrascal G, Montenegro Ramírez JD. Hygiene: basic care that promotes comfort in critically ill patients. Enferm Glob. 2015;14(4):340.
7. Al-Shamaly HS. A focused ethnography of the culture of inclusive caring practice in the intensive care unit. Nurs Open. 2021;8(6):2973–85.
8. World Health Organization, WHO Patient Safety. WHO guidelines on hand hygiene in health care. 2009;(WHO/IER/PSP/2009/01):262.
9. Davis K, Schoenbaum SC, Audet AM. A 2020 vision of patient-centered primary care. J Gen Intern Med. 2005;20(10):953–7.
10. Tunlind A, Granström J, Engström Å. Nursing care in a high-technological environment: experiences of critical care nurses. Intensive Crit Care Nurs. 2015;31(2):116–23.
11. El-Soussi AH, Asfour HI. A return to the basics; nurses' practices and knowledge about interventional patient hygiene in critical care units. Intensive Crit Care Nurs. 2017;40:11–7.
12. McGuckin M, Shubin A, Hujcs M. Interventional patient hygiene model: infection control and nursing share responsibility for patient safety. Am J Infect Control. 2008;36(1):59–62.
13. Couchman BA, Wetzig SM, Coyer FM, Wheeler MK. Nursing care of the mechanically ventilated patient: what does the evidence say? Intensive Crit Care Nurs. 2007;23(1):4–14.
14. Çelik S, Öztekin D, Akyolcu N, İşsever H. Sleep disturbance: the patient care activities applied at the night shift in the intensive care unit. J Clin Nurs. 2005;14(1):102–6.
15. Mansour W, Knauert M. Adding insult to injury. Clin Chest Med. 2022;43(2):287–303.
16. Boyko Y, Jennum P, Toft P. Sleep quality and circadian rhythm disruption in the intensive care unit: a review. Nat Sci Sleep. 2017;9:277–84.
17. Kamdar BB, Yang J, King LM, Neufeld KJ, Bienvenu OJ, Rowden AM, et al. Developing, implementing, and evaluating a multifaceted quality improvement intervention to promote sleep in an ICU. Am J Med Qual. 2014;29(6):546–54.
18. Knauert MP, Redeker NS, Yaggi HK, Bennick M, Pisani MA. Creating naptime: an overnight, nonpharmacologic intensive care unit sleep promotion protocol. J Patient Exp. 2018;5(3):180–7.

19. Tonna JE, Dalton A, Presson AP, Zhang C, Colantuoni E, Lander K, et al. The effect of a quality improvement intervention on sleep and delirium in critically ill patients in a surgical ICU. Chest. 2021;160(3):899–908.
20. Prin M, Bertazzo J, Walker LA, Scott B, Eckle T. Enhancing circadian rhythms—the circadian MEGA bundle as novel approach to treat critical illness. Ann Transl Med. 2023;11(9):319–9.
21. Anaissie EJ, Penzak SR, Dignani MC. The hospital water supply as a source of nosocomial infections: a plea for action. Arch Intern Med. 2002;162(13):1483.
22. Marchaim D, Taylor AR, Hayakawa K, Bheemreddy S, Sunkara B, Moshos J, et al. Hospital bath basins are frequently contaminated with multidrug-resistant human pathogens. Am J Infect Control. 2012;40(6):562–4.
23. Martin ET, Haider S, Palleschi M, Eagle S, Crisostomo DV, Haddox P, et al. Bathing hospitalized dependent patients with prepackaged disposable washcloths instead of traditional bath basins: a case-crossover study. Am J Infect Control. 2017;45(9):990–4.
24. Climo MW, Yokoe DS, Warren DK, Perl TM, Bolon M, Herwaldt LA, et al. Effect of daily chlorhexidine bathing on hospital-acquired infection. N Engl J Med. 2013;368(6):533–42.
25. Swan JT, Ashton CM, Bui LN, Pham VP, Shirkey BA, Blackshear JE, et al. Effect of chlorhexidine bathing every other day on prevention of hospital-acquired infections in the surgical ICU: a single-center, randomized controlled trial*. Crit Care Med. 2016;44(10):1822–32.
26. Lewis SR, Schofield-Robinson OJ, Rhodes S, Smith AF. Chlorhexidine bathing of the critically ill for the prevention of hospital-acquired infection. Cochrane Wounds Group, editor. Cochrane Database Syst Rev. 2019 [cited 2023 Nov 6]. https://doi.wiley.com/10.1002/14651858.CD012248.pub2.
27. Puntillo K, Nelson JE, Weissman D, Curtis R, Weiss S, Frontera J, et al. Palliative care in the ICU: relief of pain, dyspnea, and thirst—a report from the IPAL-ICU Advisory Board. Intensive Care Med. 2014;40(2):235–48.
28. Dale CM, Rose L, Carbone S, Pinto R, Smith OM, Burry L, et al. Effect of oral chlorhexidine de-adoption and implementation of an oral care bundle on mortality for mechanically ventilated patients in the intensive care unit (CHORAL): a multi-center stepped wedge cluster-randomized controlled trial. Intensive Care Med. 2021;47(11):1295–302.
29. Zhao T, Wu X, Zhang Q, Li C, Worthington HV, Hua F. Oral hygiene care for critically ill patients to prevent ventilator-associated pneumonia. Cochrane Oral Health Group, editor. Cochrane Database Syst Rev. 2020 [cited 2023 Nov 6];2020(12). http://doi.wiley.com/10.1002/14651858.CD008367.pub4.
30. Hearne BJ, Hearne EG, Montgomery H, Lightman SL. Eye care in the intensive care unit. J Intensive Care Soc. 2018;19(4):345–50.
31. Alansari MA, Hijazi MH, Maghrabi KA. Making a difference in eye care of the critically ill patients. J Intensive Care Med. 2015;30(6):311–7.
32. Bendavid I, Avisar I, Serov Volach I, Sternfeld A, Dan Brazis I, Umar L, et al. Prevention of exposure keratopathy in critically ill patients: a single-center, randomized, pilot trial comparing ocular lubrication with bandage contact lenses and punctal plugs. Crit Care Med. 2017;45(11):1880–6.
33. Zhou Y, Liu J, Cui Y, Zhu H, Lu Z. Moisture chamber versus lubrication for corneal protection in critically ill patients: a meta-analysis. Cornea. 2014;33(11):1179–85.
34. Treede RD. The International Association for the Study of Pain definition of pain: as valid in 2018 as in 1979, but in need of regularly updated footnotes. Pain Rep. 2018;3(2):e643.
35. Scher C, Meador L, Van Cleave JH, Reid MC. Moving beyond pain as the fifth vital sign and patient satisfaction scores to improve pain care in the 21st century. Pain Manag Nurs. 2018;19(2):125–9.
36. Luetz A, Balzer F, Radtke FM, Jones C, Citerio G, Walder B, et al. Delirium, sedation and analgesia in the intensive care unit: a multinational, two-part survey among intensivists. PLoS One. 2014;9(11):e110935.
37. Pandharipande PP, Patel MB, Barr J. Management of pain, agitation, and delirium in critically ill patients. Pol Arch Med Wewn. 2014;124(3):114–23.

38. Schelling G, Richter M, Roozendaal B, Rothenhäusler HB, Krauseneck T, Stoll C, et al. Exposure to high stress in the intensive care unit may have negative effects on health-related quality-of-life outcomes after cardiac surgery. Crit Care Med. 2003;31(7):1971–80.
39. Kyranou M, Puntillo K. The transition from acute to chronic pain: might intensive care unit patients be at risk? Ann Intensive Care. 2012;2(1):36.
40. Griffiths J, Fortune G, Barber V, Young JD. The prevalence of post traumatic stress disorder in survivors of ICU treatment: a systematic review. Intensive Care Med. 2007;33(9):1506–18.
41. Korosec Jagodic H, Jagodic K, Podbregar M. Long-term outcome and quality of life of patients treated in surgical intensive care: a comparison between sepsis and trauma. Crit Care. 2006;10(5):R134.
42. Chanques G, Sebbane M, Barbotte E, Viel E, Eledjam JJ, Jaber S. A prospective study of pain at rest: incidence and characteristics of an unrecognized symptom in surgical and trauma versus medical intensive care unit patients. Anesthesiology. 2007;107(5):858–60.
43. Barr J, Fraser GL, Puntillo K, Ely EW, Gélinas C, Dasta JF, et al. Clinical practice guidelines for the management of pain, agitation, and delirium in adult patients in the intensive care unit. Crit Care Med. 2013;41(1):263–306.
44. Vinclair M, Schilte C, Roudaud F, Lavolaine J, Francony G, Bouzat P, et al. Using pupillary pain index to assess nociception in sedated critically ill patients. Anesth Analg. 2019;129(6):1540–6.
45. Gélinas C, Tousignant-Laflamme Y, Tanguay A, Bourgault P. Exploring the validity of the bispectral index, the Critical-Care Pain Observation Tool and vital signs for the detection of pain in sedated and mechanically ventilated critically ill adults: a pilot study. Intensive Crit Care Nurs. 2011;27(1):46–52.
46. Devlin JW, Skrobik Y, Gélinas C, Needham DM, Slooter AJC, Pandharipande PP, et al. Clinical practice guidelines for the prevention and management of pain, agitation/sedation, delirium, immobility, and sleep disruption in adult patients in the ICU. Crit Care Med. 2018;46(9):e825–73.
47. Marra A, Ely EW, Pandharipande PP, Patel MB. The ABCDEF bundle in critical care. Crit Care Clin. 2017;33(2):225–43.
48. Payen JF, Bru O, Bosson JL, Lagrasta A, Novel E, Deschaux I, et al. Assessing pain in critically ill sedated patients by using a behavioral pain scale. Crit Care Med. 2001;29(12):2258–63.
49. Dale CM, Prendergast V, Gélinas C, Rose L. Validation of the Critical-care Pain Observation Tool (CPOT) for the detection of oral-pharyngeal pain in critically ill adults. J Crit Care. 2018;48:334–8.
50. Kotfis K, Zegan-Barańska M, Szydłowski Ł, Żukowski M, Ely EW. Methods of pain assessment in adult intensive care unit patients—Polish version of the CPOT (Critical Care Pain Observation Tool) and BPS (Behavioral Pain Scale). Anaesthesiol Intensive Ther. 2017;49(1):66–72.
51. Shannon K, Bucknall T. Pain assessment in critical care: what have we learnt from research. Intensive Crit Care Nurs. 2003;19(3):154–62.
52. Lindenbaum L, Milia DJ. Pain management in the ICU. Surg Clin North Am. 2012;92(6):1621–36.
53. Nishimori M, Ballantyne JC, Low JHS. Epidural pain relief versus systemic opioid-based pain relief for abdominal aortic surgery. Cochrane Database Syst Rev. 2006;(3):CD005059.
54. Schulz-Stübner S, Boezaart A, Hata JS. Regional analgesia in the critically ill. Crit Care Med. 2005;33(6):1400–7.
55. Gélinas C, Arbour C, Michaud C, Robar L, Côté J. Patients and ICU nurses' perspectives of non-pharmacological interventions for pain management. Nurs Crit Care. 2013;18(6):307–18.
56. Umbreit AW. Healing touch: applications in the acute care setting. AACN Clin Issues Adv Pract Acute Crit Care. 2000;11(1):105–19.
57. Morse JM, Bottorff JL, Hutchinson S. The phenomenology of comfort. J Adv Nurs. 1994;20(1):189–95.

58. Seyffert S, Moiz S, Coghlan M, Balozian P, Nasser J, Rached EA, et al. Decreasing delirium through music listening (DDM) in critically ill, mechanically ventilated older adults in the intensive care unit: a two-arm, parallel-group, randomized clinical trial. Trials. 2022;23(1):576.

59. Yue W, Han X, Luo J, Zeng Z, Yang M. Effect of music therapy on preterm infants in neonatal intensive care unit: systematic review and meta-analysis of randomized controlled trials. J Adv Nurs. 2021;77(2):635–52.

60. Rousseaux F, Faymonville ME, Nyssen AS, Dardenne N, Ledoux D, Massion PB, et al. Can hypnosis and virtual reality reduce anxiety, pain and fatigue among patients who undergo cardiac surgery: a randomised controlled trial. Trials. 2020;21(1):330.

61. Naef AC, Gerber SM, Single M, Müri RM, Haenggi M, Jakob SM, et al. Effects of immersive virtual reality on sensory overload in a random sample of critically ill patients. Front Med. 2023;10:1268659.

62. Merliot-Gailhoustet L, Raimbert C, Garnier O, Carr J, De Jong A, Molinari N, et al. Discomfort improvement for critically ill patients using electronic relaxation devices: results of the cross-over randomized controlled trial E-CHOISIR (Electronic-CHOIce of a System for Intensive care Relaxation). Crit Care. 2022;26(1):263.

Nutrition: One Size Does Not Fit All

4

Judith L. Merriweather

4.1 Introduction

With increasing ICU survival, the physical, emotional and psychological complications of critical illness are increasingly recognised. This constellation of health-related morbidities is summarised under the term 'post-intensive care syndrome' (PICS). PICS is an internationally recognised concept of stepwise deterioration in physical, psychological and cognitive status following ICU discharge [1]. Nutrition plays an important role in managing or mitigating features of PICS, with the maintenance of nutritional health essential for optimal physiological, physical and psychological functioning. There are many factors which impact on nutritional status during the critical illness trajectory, and these are discussed in more detail below.

4.2 Presence of Pre-existing Conditions on Admission to ICU

4.2.1 Chronic Co-morbidities

Critically ill patients are a highly heterogeneous population who tend to have many chronic comorbid medical conditions such as cardiovascular disease, diabetes, chronic obstructive pulmonary disease, malignancies, liver disease and/or obesity [2]. These chronic disease states have been shown to have similar pathophysiological features resulting in low-grade inflammation [3]. Multiple

J. L. Merriweather (✉)
The Royal Infirmary of Edinburgh, NHS Lothian, Edinburgh, UK

The University of Edinburgh, Edinburgh, UK
e-mail: Judith.Merriweather@ed.ac.uk

C. Boulanger, D. McWilliams (eds.), *Passport to Successful Outcomes for Patients Admitted to ICU*, https://doi.org/10.1007/978-3-031-53019-7_4

49

studies have observed associations between inflammatory markers and muscle protein breakdown, resulting in muscle wasting and reduced muscle function [4].

4.2.2 Sarcopenia

Sarcopenia, a condition characterised by progressive and generalised loss of muscle mass, occurs as a primary consequence of ageing [5]. The literature suggests that the prevalence of sarcopenia in 60 to 70-year-olds is in the range of 5–13% [6]. National data show that there are increasing numbers of elderly patients being admitted to ICUs, increasing the likelihood of sarcopenia-related muscle mass loss in ICU populations. As muscle loss is an identified feature of malnutrition [7], it is probable that many patients admitted to ICU are at high risk of developing malnutrition.

4.2.3 Malnutrition

The prevalence of malnutrition on admission to ICU has been reported as 43% of general ICU admissions [8]. It is important to note that the length of hospital stay and the incidence of complications were greater in the malnourished group. Other studies using a different tool to assess nutritional status found that 23–54% of patients admitted to ICU are moderately to severely malnourished [9]. A recent systematic review found the pooled prevalence of malnutrition risk in COVID 19 ICU patients was as high as 92% [10]. Malnourished patients have a higher mortality rates and increased rates of ICU readmission [11]. Low muscle mass, which is associated with malnutrition, has been identified in 63% of patients admitted to a medical ICU [12]. Low skeletal muscle area was associated with increased mortality.

4.3 Factors Which Affect Nutritional Status During ICU Stay

4.3.1 Metabolic Response to Critical Illness

The onset of acute illness is characterised by a metabolic response involving a neuroendocrine and an inflammatory/immune component. Triggering the neuroendocrine pathway results in stimulation of the sympathetic nervous system and the hypothalamic–pituitary–adrenal axis [13]. The resulting elevations in cortisol, glucagon and catecholamines evoke a number of metabolic consequences that affect energy, protein and fat metabolism. The inflammatory response results in the release of cytokines and immune mediators, which directly and indirectly exert a number of metabolic effects [14].

This complex metabolic response results in altered energy production pathways characterised by excessive gluconeogenesis, glycogenolysis and insulin resistance, which results in hyperglycaemia [15]. Recent practice has focused on the effects of hyperglycaemia and its treatment [16]; however, hypertriglyceridemia and protein breakdown are also major consequences of insulin resistance [17]. Although insulin resistance is considered an adaptive mechanism that provides sufficient amounts of glucose to the vital organs unable to use other energy substrates in stress conditions [13], there are significant consequences of hyperglycaemia, hypertriglyceridemia and protein breakdown, all having an impact on recovery.

The clinical consequences of the metabolic response to stress include alterations to metabolic rate, use of macronutrients as a source of energy, stress hyperglycaemia, loss of muscle mass and changes in body composition [14]. These features were particularly evident in critically ill patients with COVID-19 who were found to experience prolonged hypermetabolism, sustained proinflammatory state and consequent catabolic effects [18].

4.3.2   Iatrogenic Undernutrition

Nutritional support is instigated early in critical illness aiming to attenuate catabolism and preserve lean body mass [19]. However in ICU, nutrition delivery is largely inadequate with mechanically ventilated patients characteristically only receiving 60–70% of their prescribed protein and energy requirements [20, 21]. This suboptimal intake results from delays in initiating feeding [22], feed interruptions due to nausea, vomiting, abdominal distension, large gastric aspirates, tube displacement, investigations and prolonged fasting for procedures [21]. Consequently, over the course of their ICU stay, critically ill patients accrue large energy and protein deficits [23] which are associated with a reduction in ventilator-free days, increased ICU and hospital length of stay [24].

4.3.3   Immobilisation

Malnutrition and muscle wasting generally occur during ICU stay due to the effect of catabolic hormones, an imbalance between intake and requirements and also as a result of physical immobilisation. Large amounts of lean body mass as well as fat mass may be lost during a relatively short time during an ICU stay [25]. Low mechanical load induced by bed rest, immobilisation and muscle disuse results in not only a significant reduction in muscle mass but also loss of muscle strength and physiological function [26]. A complex cytokine and inflammatory response, initiated by immobility, results in muscle proteolysis promoting overall muscle loss [25]. This loss of muscle can be considered as frailty, a concept usually associated with the elderly [27]. However, parallels have been drawn with the critically ill patient where frailty is characterised by adverse changes to a patient's mobility, muscle mass and nutritional status [28].

Ultimately, all these factors lead to changes in body composition in critically ill patients. Puthucheary [28] examined the loss of muscle over the first 7 days of ICU admission. Ultrasound measurements of rectus femoris cross-sectional area (CSA) showed the greatest reduction in CSA in patients who experienced multiple organ failure compared with single organ failure by day 7 (−15.7% [95% CI, −19.1% to −12.4%] vs. −3.0% [95% CI, −10.5% to 4.6%], P <0.001). Other studies looking at changes in body composition found that the rate of weight loss and muscle wasting is highest in the first 2 weeks of admission to ICU, with sicker patients experiencing the highest [29]. A seminal study by Herridge et al. [30] explored weight loss over the whole critical illness trajectory. Survivors of acute respiratory distress syndrome were found to have lost 18% of their baseline body weight on discharge from ICU, with muscle weakness and fatigue cited as the reasons for functional limitation. It has long been recognised that muscle wasting in critical illness has implications for recovery and rehabilitation and is associated with a reduction in functional capacity, quality of life and prolonged hospital stay.

4.4   Assessing Malnutrition in the Critically Ill Patient

Currently, there is no consensus on how to diagnose malnutrition in the critically ill with body composition and physical and functional impairments measured using a variety of different tools [26, 31]. Weight changes are difficult to determine in the ICU due to the presence of oedema, fluid shifts and rapid muscle wasting. Therefore, weight and body mass index (BMI), commonly used in the hospital to assess nutritional status, do not accurately reflect malnutrition in critically ill patients.

4.4.1   Nutrition Screening Tools

A number of nutritional assessment tools have been used in the intensive care setting, although no specific ICU nutritional score has been validated thus far. Subjective Global Assessment (SGA) is used to assess nutritional status and is based on physical assessment of muscle and fat stores, history of nutrition intake, weight changes, identification of symptoms influencing oral intake and the presence of illness that may alter metabolic demands [32]. Sheean [9] compared SGA with three other commonly used tools: the Mini Nutrition Assessment (MNA), Nutrition Risk Screening and MNA-Short Form (MNA-SF). Results showed that compared to MNA, NRS 2002 had the highest sensitivity, while SGA and MNA-SF had higher specificity.

NUTRIC, a novel tool that was designed to categorise nutrition risk, was proposed by the American Society for Parenteral and Enteral (ASPEN)/Society for Critical Care Medicine (SCCM) [19] to determine nutritional therapy. This tool assessed nutritional risk based on age, severity of disease, co-morbidities, number of days from hospital to ICU admission and including or excluding the presence of inflammation with the cumulative scores correlated with mortality. The recent ESPEN guideline on clinical nutrition in the intensive care unit disagreed with this recommendation, as no nutritional parameters are included in the score. A comparison of NUTRIC with traditional screening tools found large variations [31].

The ESPEN guidelines [31] suggest that in the absence of a validated screening tool for ICU patients, a general clinical assessment should be performed to assess malnutrition. The guidance recommends adopting a pragmatic approach when considering at-risk patients to include patients in ICU >2 days; mechanically ventilated; suboptimal oral intake >5 days; presence of infection and/or presenting with a severe chronic disease.

4.4.2 Muscle Mass

Other methods have been used in ICU to determine lean body mass loss including mid-upper arm circumference (MUAC), bioelectrical impedance analysis (BIA), ultrasound or computed tomography (CT) scan. MUAC has been shown to be simple and feasible to measure in the ICU and may have prognostic value in identifying those most at nutritional risk when values are compared with population norms [33].

BIA can be used to assess body composition; however, the use of the raw BIA parameter, phase angle (PhA), avoids algorithm-inherent errors and the need for constant tissue [34]. PhA has been shown to be a useful tool in identifying nutritional risk and prognosis of critically ill patients.

Muscle ultrasound has been shown to predict lean body mass as accurately as magnetic resonance imaging (MRI) or CT [35]. This technology has been shown to have excellent inter-rater and intra-rater reliability when performed by a variety of health care professionals [36].

Recently, CT scan has been used to assess lean body mass and has been shown to be precise, reliable and is a promising tool for identifying patients who may benefit from targeted nutritional interventions [29]; however, its use is limited to those requiring CT scans as part of routine care.

A systematic review identified at least 33 different measures of skeletal muscle mass, strength and function for use in critically ill patients [37]. The most appropriate measure to be used at each stage of the critical care journey is currently unknown; however, what is clear is that recovery in ICU survivors is poor, with functional deficits still present 5 years after ICU discharge [38].

4.5 Strategies to Improve Physical and Functional Outcomes

Mortality has been predominately used as a primary outcome measure, in large prospective randomised controlled trials (RCTs) of nutrition in the critically ill [39]. More recently, however, with increased recognition of the functional disability associated with survivorship, there has been a shift in emphasis towards the physical and functional recovery of ICU survivors. The need for this shift became particularly evident during the pandemic when critical illness secondary to COVID-19 produced an overwhelming surge in ICU admissions with survivors experiencing a range of physical and functional deficits.

There are a number of factors which need to be taken into consideration when looking at nutritional interventions such as amount of nutrients to be delivered, timing and route of administration. Nutrition studies in critical care have examined the nutrition administered to the patient, not what is actually delivered relative to requirements.

The average length of stay for critically ill patients is around a week, and the majority of nutrition interventions in RCTs are only administered for 6–7 days which is unlikely to result in a measurable effect on the outcome. This was demonstrated in the TARGET trial where providing 30.2 kcal/kg/day versus 21.9 kcal/kg/day over a median period of 6 days had no effect on outcomes in any subgroup [40]. Another large RCT, EAT-ICU failed to show any demonstrable benefit of delivering a 7-day nutrition intervention on the physical quality of life at 6 months after randomisation [41].

4.5.1 Targeted Nutrition Delivery

Nutritional needs change over the course of critical illness. It is well recognised that the acute phase of critical illness is associated with substrate mobilisation as muscle, glycogen and fat are broken down to drive glucose production [42]. This catabolic response can generate 50–75% of glucose requirements during the initial few days in ICU [14]. As there is no bedside method currently available to measure endogenous energy production, it is impossible to account for this when calculating energy expenditure. In line with this, the ESPEN guidelines [31] recommended energy goals should be achieved progressively over the first 1–4 days of ICU admission. The results from two recent RCTs continue to support the ESPEN guideline recommendation for hypocaloric feeding during the early phase of critical illness [43, 44].

In the later stage of critical illness, endogenous energy stores have been depleted and energy expenditure markedly increases although currently there are a lack of objective measures for determining when a patient shifts from the acute phase to the recovery phase. During this recovery phase, the demand for exogenous energy will be increased for anabolic purposes [45]. The use of indirect calorimetry to measure energy expenditure to determine energy goals has been recommended instead of predictive equations, as their use can result in significant under- or overfeeding [46]. With the advent of more affordable calorimeters designed specifically for critically ill patients, it should facilitate research into the effect of targeted energy feeding on physical and functional recovery.

4.5.2 Volume-Based Feeding

Despite the need to ensure optimal nutritional intake, critically ill patients do not meet the recommended energy and protein targets. Data from an observational cohort study of nutrition practices in ICUs across 37 countries have shown that critically ill patients receive a daily average of 1034 kcal and 47 g protein over the first 12 days of their ICU stay [47]. The duration of hypocaloric feeding is far longer than the recommended 1–4 days, which may have a detrimental effect on nutritional status and lead to longer term issues, with reduced physical function in ICU survivors.

As previously highlighted, enteral nutrient delivery is often impaired by gastrointestinal intolerance or prolonged fasting for a variety of procedures [21]. Historically, feeding practices in ICU were based on an hourly rate-based feeding (RBF) approach; however more recently, a volume-based feeding approach (VBF) has been suggested. This approach is designed to adjust the infusion rate to make up for daily interruptions in delivery, enabling a greater volume of EN to be delivered compared to a fixed hourly RBF. Findings from an RCT showed that VBF resulted in 12–15% increase in the amount of protein and calories received by the patient [48]. Although a number of studies have shown improvements in nutrient delivery with VBF, not all have shown improved outcomes when energy and protein goals are achieved. Some have shown no significant difference in length of stay (LOS), mortality or ventilation days with volume-based feeding; others have demonstrated a reduction in mortality, ventilation and LOS when energy and protein targets are met [49]. As there has been limited focus on muscle wasting and functional performance as outcomes in critical care nutrition trials, the effects of VBF on these outcomes remain unclear.

4.5.3 Energy Versus Protein

Another question that needs to be addressed is the importance of protein delivery to improve outcome in the ICU. The majority of nutrition trials in critical care have focussed on the provision of energy, particularly during the first week of ICU stay, and not on the amount of protein that was delivered. A number of observational studies have shown improved outcomes and reduced muscle mass loss when increased protein is delivered [12, 50, 51]. Current ESPEN guidance [31] recommends a protein intake of 1.3 g/kg/day delivered progressively. However, meta-analysis showed high protein was not associated with improvements in clinical or patient-centred outcomes [52], and the recent EFFORT trial found no benefit from higher protein doses (>2.2 g/kg/day) [53]. Subgroup analysis of this trial suggests worse outcomes with high protein doses for patients with acute kidney injury who were not on renal replacement therapy and those with high admitting sequential organ failure assessment (SOFA) score.

There is also conflicting evidence surrounding the optimal timing of protein provision. Some researchers advocate early protein administration [12, 51]; however, findings from a retrospective study found that high protein intake, during the first few days of ICU stay, was associated with increased mortality [54].

There is a need for RCTs to determine the optimal dose and timing of protein administration based on individual patient characteristics in ICU to enhance muscle strength and function. Further sub-studies from the EFFORT trial are currently underway to explore the effect of higher dose of protein on muscle mass and physical functional recovery.

4.5.4 Exercise and Protein

In the absence of any pharmacological intervention to prevent muscle loss, two important stimuli are exercise and protein delivery. It is the combination of exercise and amino acid delivery that results in muscle protein synthesis, and this has been demonstrated in various patient populations including the elderly, obese, HIV and chronic obstructive pulmonary disease. In a meta-analysis, protein supplementation with exercise, compared with exercise alone, increased muscle mass and strength in healthy subjects [55]. Administration of increased protein intake, together with increased activity in the ICU, should be further explored; however, it will require circumventing factors which may influence functional ability including fatigue, pain, delirium and the patients' pre-illness health and age [56].

4.5.5   Supplementation

B-Hydroxy-β-methylbutyrate (HMB) has been shown to be an effective pharmaconutrient in the modulation of muscle mass, resulting in increased muscle protein synthesis and reduced muscle protein breakdown in healthy adults. A systematic review and meta-analysis HMB and supplements containing HMB were found to increase muscle mass and strength in a variety of clinical conditions including COPD, cancer and malnutrition, although the effect size was small. The authors concluded that given the bias associated with many of the studies, further high-quality studies were required to facilitate translation into clinical practice [57]. Two recent HMB studies in ICU populations reported no difference in muscle loss [58, 59], although it is possible the intervention period was too short to be of benefit [60].

4.6   Recovery Phase of Critical Illness

Despite the fact that ICU survivors frequently suffer significant prolonged physical disability, especially those with prolonged ventilation or significant multi-organ failure, there are few studies investigating the influence of nutritional support beyond the first 7 days of critical illness, or indeed the extent of malnutrition at the time of extubation. However, it is highly likely that critically ill patients, with a higher severity of illness and prolonged ventilation, will be malnourished during the latter stages of their ICU stay.

In the aftermath of the COVID-19 pandemic, where the need for rehabilitation for COVID-19 ICU survivors was amplified, it is clear that further research is needed to improve long term functional outcomes. Research in the role of nutrition in the recovery phase of critical illness remains scarce and existing post-ICU nutritional rehabilitation strategies fail to address the functional limitations experienced by ICU survivors [61]. Current knowledge of post ICU nutrition is based on small observational studies. These studies have focussed primarily on two main themes: the adequacy of nutrient delivery and the factors that influence nutritional recovery.

Table 4.1 Energy and protein intakes in patients after extubation

	Route of feeding	Adequacy of caloric intake (%)	Adequacy of protein intake (%)
Peterson et al. [62][a] n = 50	Oral nutrition	35–55	23–37
Chapple et al. [23][b] n = 37	EN alone	89	76
	Oral nutrition (food only)	75	74
Ridley et al. [63][c] n = 32	EN alone	62 [21–96]	59 [20.5–97]
	Oral nutrition (food only)	66 [38–89]	60 [37–83]
	Oral nutrition (food and supplements)	37 [21–66]	48 [13–63]
	EN and oral nutrition combined	73 [51–94] 104 [66–132]	68 [49–84] 99 [60–127]
Wittholz et al. [64][b] n = 28	Oral nutrition	54	65
	EN, EN and oral diet, PN	87	87
Moisey et al. [65][b] n = 19	Oral nutrition	47	27
	EN alone	100	100
	EN and oral nutrition combined	74	75

[a] Data are presented as a range of means
[b] Data are presented as a mean
[c] Data are presented as median [interquartile range]

4.7   Adequacy of Nutrient Delivery

To date, there are a number of small studies which have quantified energy and protein intakes in patients after extubation (Table 4.1). One study of 50 patients from a medical/surgical ICU found that energy and protein intakes were less than 55% and 37% of requirements, respectively, during the first 7 days following extubation [62]. Chapple et al. [23] evaluated the nutritional intake of 37 traumatic brain injury patients and found those on oral diets consumed 75% and 74% of their energy and protein requirements, whereas those receiving enteral nutrition received 89% and 75% of their estimated energy and protein requirements. Ridey et al. collected nutritional data from 32 patients during their post-ICU hospitalisation period. Findings showed that patients on oral diet alone met only 66% and 60% of their nutritional requirements, with those on a combination of diet and enteral nutrition achieving 104% and 99% of energy and protein requirements [63]. Wittholz et al. [64] explored the nutritional intakes of 28 trauma patients following discharge from ICU and found patients receiving oral diets consumed a mean of 54% and 65% of prescribed calories and protein, respectively. Adequacy of calorie and protein intake for patients receiving artificial nutrition (EN, EN with an oral diet, PN) was 87% and 87%, respectively. In the most recent study Moisey et al. [65] assessed nutritional intakes of 19 patients from a medical/surgical ICU over the first 14 days post extubation. Findings showed patients receiving oral diets consumed median 47% and 27% of prescribed calories and protein, respectively. The adequacy of calorie and protein intake for patients on EN and

Table 4.2 Themes and sub themes influencing the nutritional recovery process

Themes	Experiencing a dysfunctional body	Experiencing sociocultural changes in relation to eating	Encountering organisational nutritional care delivery failures
Sub-themes	Facing physiological changes	Experiencing social isolation	Experiencing system-centred failures
	Facing psychological changes	Struggling to adapt to an unfamiliar culture	Struggling with an inflexible hospital routine
	Dealing with changes to body, self and identity	Importance of food habits and routine	Communication failures Staff knowledge gap

EN with an oral diet was 100% and 100%, respectively, and 74% and 75%, respectively.

As this is an under-researched area, no guidelines exist for the nutritional care of the ICU patient following extubation. Further research is required to clarify the nutritional targets, optimal route of nutrient delivery and timings for transitioning from enteral to oral nutrition in ICU survivors.

4.7.1 Factors Influencing Nutritional Recovery

From the few studies that have looked at nutritional intakes in patients after extubation, it is clear that patients fail to meet their nutritional requirements, particularly with oral diet alone. Qualitative work has identified multiple factors that contributed to patients' failure to achieve nutritional goals (Table 4.2) [66].

The identified factors that influence nutritional recovery interlink, serving to increase the complexity of nutritional problems for this patient group.

4.8 Potential Strategies to Facilitate Optimal Nutritional Delivery in the Recovery Phase of Critical Illness

4.8.1 Coordinated Multidisciplinary Approach to Nutritional Care

A consistent, systematic approach to the management of the identified physiological factors influencing nutritional intake such as nausea, vomiting and diarrhoea is required. A number of studies have identified that early removal of ng tubes is associated with a reduction in nutritional intake [66–68] These data suggest that prolonged tube feeding until oral nutrition intake is sufficient should be considered as an alternative to usual care. If a patient is malnourished on admission to ICU, is likely to have a protracted ICU stay or has a diagnosis that is associated with nutritional issues, e.g. pancreatitis, then consideration should be given to the most appropriate route for feeding, taking into account the longer term nutritional issues that these patients are likely to face. A multidisciplinary team discussion could identify patients who would benefit from the placement of longer term feeding tubes in order to facilitate effective nutritional care in ICU, and after transfer to the ward.

Similarly, a multidisciplinary team approach would be beneficial in the discussion of patients who were ready for discharge to the ward. Patients with ongoing or complex issues could be identified and where possible, out-of-hours transfers avoided. It has been shown that patients who were transferred out of hours experienced more nutritional issues on the ward such as removal of ng tubes or failure to deliver nutritional supplements [67].

4.8.2 Systematic Handover to Ward-Based Staff

A clearly documented nutritional management plan should be handed over to ward staff and appropriate allied health professionals to include any issues influencing nutritional intake in ICU, e.g. physiological factors such as poor appetite, early satiety, taste changes, weakness, fatigue or psychological issues such as low mood or delirium. Other information on the management plan should include a description of the patient's current nutritional intake, incorporating nutrition from parenteral, enteral and oral routes, food likes and dislikes and details about family involvement in nutritional care. Finally, the plan for ongoing nutritional care should be clearly described. Specific recommendations should be clearly communicated, to reduce ill-informed decision-making by ward-based staff. These recommendations may include the need to continue with enteral feeding or nutritional supplements.

4.8.3 Patient Centred Nutritional Care and Family Engagement

The provision of nutritional care on the ward has traditionally taken a service centred approach where care is organised around the service and not the patient. To better meet the needs of ICU survivors, it is suggested that a patient-centred approach should be adopted to promote patient autonomy, shared decision making and feedback from the patient [69]. As part of this approach, the patient and family will require education about nutritional needs in the recovery phase of critical illness with information and feedback provided on achieving nutritional targets. Guidance should be given about the types of food family members could bring in, such as energy-dense, protein-rich snacks to optimise nutritional intakes. This involvement of the family helps create a culture that 'acknowledges and values the importance of this patient-family-nurse interaction' [70].

A patient pathway has been devised to define the key elements of nutritional care for ICU survivors during each of the three stages of care: prior to transfer from ICU, during ward stay and on discharge from hospital (Table 4.3).

Table 4.3 Pathway to promote the provision of effective nutritional care for ICU survivors

Prior to discharge from the intensive care unit	
Goal 1: The patient's nutritional issues are identified early	• Pre-existing malnutrition prior to ICU admission (BMI < 18 kg m², history of weight loss and/or history of poor nutritional intake) • Long ICU stay (>7 days) • Swallowing problems Patient experiencing physiological factors influencing nutritional intake 　• Loss of appetite 　• Early satiety 　• Taste changes 　• Pain 　• Nausea/vomiting 　• Diarrhoea 　• Fatigue 　• Breathlessness 　• Changes to sleep patterns Patient experiencing psychological factors influencing nutritional intake 　• Delirium 　• Low mood 　• Cognitive changes 　• Depression
Goal 2: The patient's identified nutritional issues are communicated to ward staff	Handover to ward staff to include: 　• Current route for nutrition 　• Identified factors influencing nutritional intake 　• Nutritional plan
During ward stay	
Goal 3: The patient is receiving the appropriate amount and type of nutrition	• Weekly weights • Review by dietitian • Referral to speech and language therapy (if necessary) • Food record charts
Goal 4: The patient's ongoing physiological issues are identified	• Loss of appetite • Early satiety • Taste changes • Pain • Nausea/vomiting • Diarrhoea • Fatigue • Breathlessness • Changes to sleep patterns Issues are discussed with multidisciplinary team
Goal 5: The patient's ongoing psychological issues are identified	• Delirium • Low mood • Cognitive changes • Depression Issues are discussed with multidisciplinary team

Table 4.3 (continued)

Prior to discharge from the intensive care unit	
Goal 6: The patient has the appropriate provision of food	• Meals served one course at a time • Meals provided at suitable times • Family encouraged to bring in favourite foods • Provision of meals from canteen where necessary • Additional snacks are provided between meals • Assistance with eating is provided where necessary • Eating with others is encouraged
Goal 7: The patient is aware of the importance of good nutrition	• Emphasising the need to eat more for physical recovery • Discussion of factors affecting nutritional intake • Regular feedback to patient about adequacy of oral intake • Involvement of family in discussions
Goal 8: The patient's nutritional needs are discussed regularly by the multidisciplinary team (MDT)	• Weekly multidisciplinary meetings • Dietitian highlights any nutritional issues • The need for nutritional support is reviewed by the MDT
On discharge from hospital	
Goal 9: The patient is provided with appropriate nutritional information and aftercare	• Written dietary information • Contact details • Supply of nutritional supplements provided (if necessary) • Plan for follow-up

4.8.4 Conclusion

It is well recognised that nutritional status, particularly muscle mass deteriorates during an ICU stay, and therefore appropriate nutrition support during critical illness should be considered a necessary therapy. An individualised approach to ICU nutrition is essential and there is a need for objective data to measure nutrition needs. With the shifting focus to survivorship after critical illness, exemplified by the COVID-19 pandemic, more research is needed to ascertain the impact of nutritional interventions on physical and functional recovery.

Key Take Home Messages
- There are many factors which affect nutritional status over the critical illness trajectory.
- Nutritional assessment should be undertaken to assess malnutrition in the ICU.
- Individualised nutrition support should be provided across the continuum of care including the post-ICU phase.
- Future research should focus on innovative nutrition interventions during and after critical illness that have the potential to benefit physical and functional recovery.

References

1. Needham DM, Davidson J, Cohen H, Hopkins RO, Weinert C, Wunsch H, et al. Improving long-term outcomes after discharge from intensive care unit: report from a stakeholders' conference. Crit Care Med. 2012;40(2):502–9.
2. Esper AM, Martin GS. The impact of comorbid [corrected] conditions on critical illness. Crit Care Med. 2011;39(12):2728–35.
3. Hotamisligil GS. Inflammation and metabolic disorders. Nature. 2006;444(7121):860–7.
4. Schaap LA, Pluijm SM, Deeg DJ, Visser M. Inflammatory markers and loss of muscle mass (sarcopenia) and strength. Am J Med. 2006;119(6):526.e9–17.
5. Kizilarslanoglu MC, Kuyumcu ME, Yesil Y, Halil M. Sarcopenia in critically ill patients. J Anesth. 2016;30(5):884–90.
6. Wang C, Bai L. Sarcopenia in the elderly: basic and clinical issues. Geriatr Gerontol Int. 2012;12(3):388–96.
7. Jensen GL, Bistrian B, Roubenoff R, Heimburger DC. Malnutrition syndromes: a conundrum vs continuum. JPEN J Parenter Enteral Nutr. 2009;33(6):710–6.
8. Giner M, Laviano A, Meguid MM, Gleason JR. In 1995 a correlation between malnutrition and poor outcome in critically ill patients still exists. Nutrition. 1996;12(1):23–9.
9. Sheean PM, Peterson SJ, Chen Y, Liu D, Lateef O, Braunschweig CA. Utilizing multiple methods to classify malnutrition among elderly patients admitted to the medical and surgical intensive care units (ICU). Clin Nutr. 2013;32(5):752–7.
10. Feng X, Liu Z, He X, Wang X, Yuan C, Huang L, Song R, Wu Y. Risk of malnutrition in hospitalized COVID-19 patients: a systematic review and meta-analysis. Nutrients. 2022;14(24):5267.
11. Fontes D, Generoso Sde V, Toulson Davisson Correia MI. Subjective global assessment: a reliable nutritional assessment tool to predict outcomes in critically ill patients. Clin Nutr. 2014;33(2):291–5.
12. Weijs PJ, Looijaard WG, Beishuizen A, Girbes AR, Oudemans-van Straaten HM. Early high protein intake is associated with low mortality and energy overfeeding with high mortality in non-septic mechanically ventilated critically ill patients. Crit Care. 2014;18(6):701.
13. Marik PE, Bellomo R. Stress hyperglycemia: an essential survival response! Crit Care. 2013;17(2):305.
14. Preiser JC, Ichai C, Orban JC, Groeneveld AB. Metabolic response to the stress of critical illness. Br J Anaesth. 2014;113(6):945–54.
15. Weissman C. The metabolic response to stress: an overview and update. Anesthesiology. 1990;73(2):308–27.
16. Van den Berghe G, Wilmer A, Milants I, Wouters PJ, Bouckaert B, Bruyninckx F, et al. Intensive insulin therapy in mixed medical/surgical intensive care units: benefit versus harm. Diabetes. 2006;55(11):3151–9.
17. Dhar A, Castillo L. Insulin resistance in critical illness. Curr Opin Pediatr. 2011;23(3):269–74.
18. Whittle J, Molinger J, MacLeod D, Haines C, Wischmeyer PE, LEEP-COVID Study Group. Persistent hypermetabolism and longitudinal energy expenditure in critically ill patients with COVID-19. Crit Care. 2020;24(1):581.
19. McClave SA, Taylor BE, Martindale RG, Warren MM, Johnson DR, Braunschweig C, et al. Guidelines for the provision and assessment of nutrition support therapy in the adult critically ill patient: Society of Critical Care Medicine (SCCM) and American Society for Parenteral and Enteral Nutrition (A.S.P.E.N.). JPEN J Parenter Enteral Nutr. 2016;40(2):159–211.
20. Cahill NE, Dhaliwal R, Day AG, Jiang X, Heyland DK. Nutrition therapy in the critical care setting: what is "best achievable" practice? An international multicenter observational study. Crit Care Med. 2010;38(2):395–401.
21. Heyland DK, Dhaliwal R, Wang M, Day AG. The prevalence of iatrogenic underfeeding in the nutritionally 'at-risk' critically ill patient: results of an international, multicenter, prospective study. Clin Nutr. 2015;34(4):659–66.

22. Wandrag L, Gordon F, O'Flynn J, Siddiqui B, Hickson M. Identifying the factors that influence energy deficit in the adult intensive care unit: a mixed linear model analysis. J Hum Nutr Diet. 2011;24(3):215–22.
23. Chapple LS, Deane AM, Heyland DK, Lange K, Kranz AJ, Williams LT, et al. Energy and protein deficits throughout hospitalization in patients admitted with a traumatic brain injury. Clin Nutr. 2016;35(6):1315–22.
24. Yeh DD, Fuentes E, Quraishi SA, Cropano C, Kaafarani H, Lee J, et al. Adequate nutrition may get you home: effect of caloric/protein deficits on the discharge destination of critically ill surgical patients. JPEN J Parenter Enteral Nutr. 2016;40(1):37–44.
25. Topp R, Ditmyer M, King K, Doherty K, Hornyak J III. The effect of bed rest and potential of prehabilitation on patients in the intensive care unit. AACN Clin Issues. 2002;13(2):263–76.
26. Parry SM, Puthucheary ZA. The impact of extended bed rest on the musculoskeletal system in the critical care environment. Extrem Physiol Med. 2015;4:16.
27. Rockwood K, Song X, MacKnight C, Bergman H, Hogan DB, McDowell I, et al. A global clinical measure of fitness and frailty in elderly people. CMAJ. 2005;173(5):489–95.
28. Puthucheary ZA, Rawal J, McPhail M, Connolly B, Ratnayake G, Chan P, et al. Acute skeletal muscle wasting in critical illness. JAMA. 2013;310(15):1591–600.
29. Braunschweig CA, Sheean PM, Peterson SJ, Gomez Perez S, Freels S, Troy KL, et al. Exploitation of diagnostic computed tomography scans to assess the impact of nutrition support on body composition changes in respiratory failure patients. JPEN J Parenter Enteral Nutr. 2014;38(7):880–5.
30. Herridge MS, Cheung AM, Tansey CM, Matte-Martyn A, Diaz-Granados N, Al-Saidi F, et al. One-year outcomes in survivors of the acute respiratory distress syndrome. N Engl J Med. 2003;348(8):683–93.
31. Singer P, Blaser AR, Berger MM, Alhazzani W, Calder PC, Casaer MP, et al. ESPEN guideline on clinical nutrition in the intensive care unit. Clin Nutr. 2019;38(1):48–79.
32. Detsky AS, McLaughlin JR, Baker JP, Johnston N, Whittaker S, Mendelson RA, et al. What is subjective global assessment of nutritional status? JPEN J Parenter Enteral Nutr. 1987;11(1):8–13.
33. Ravasco P, Camilo ME, Gouveia-Oliveira A, Adam S, Brum G. A critical approach to nutritional assessment in critically ill patients. Clin Nutr. 2002;21(1):73–7.
34. Norman K, Stobaus N, Pirlich M, Bosy-Westphal A. Bioelectrical phase angle and impedance vector analysis—clinical relevance and applicability of impedance parameters. Clin Nutr. 2012;31(6):854–61.
35. Mourtzakis M, Wischmeyer P. Bedside ultrasound measurement of skeletal muscle. Curr Opin Clin Nutr Metab Care. 2014;17(5):389–95.
36. Tillquist M, Kutsogiannis DJ, Wischmeyer PE, Kummerlen C, Leung R, Stollery D, et al. Bedside ultrasound is a practical and reliable measurement tool for assessing quadriceps muscle layer thickness. JPEN J Parenter Enteral Nutr. 2014;38(7):886–90.
37. Selina M, Parry Catherine L, Granger Sue, Berney Jennifer, Jones Lisa, Beach Doa, El-Ansary René, Koopman Linda, Denehy. Assessment of impairment and activity limitations in the critically ill: a systematic review of measurement instruments and their clinimetric properties Intensive Care Medicine. 2015;41(5):744–762. https://doi.org/10.1007/s00134-015-3672-x.
38. Herridge MS, Tansey CM, Matte A, Tomlinson G, Diaz-Granados N, Cooper A, et al. Functional disability 5 years after acute respiratory distress syndrome. N Engl J Med. 2011;364(14):1293–304.
39. Taverny G, Lescot T, Pardo E, Thonon F, Maarouf M, Alberti C. Outcomes used in randomised controlled trials of nutrition in the critically ill: a systematic review. Crit Care. 2019;23(1):12.
40. Target Investigators for the ANZICS Clinical Trials Group, Chapman M, Peake SL, Bellomo R, Davies A, Deane A, et al. Energy-dense versus routine enteral nutrition in the critically ill. N Engl J Med. 2018;379(19):1823–34.
41. Allingstrup MJ, Kondrup J, Wils J, Claudius C, Pedersen UG, Hein-Rasmussen R, et al. Early goal-directed nutrition versus standard of care in adult intensive care patients: the single centre, randomised, outcome assessor-blinded EAT-ICU trial. Intensive Care Med. 2017;43:1637–47.

42. Gillis C, Carli F. Promoting perioperative metabolic and nutritional care. Anesthesiology. 2015;123(6):1455–72.
43. Pardo E, Lescot T, Preiser JC, Massanet P, Pons A, Jaber S, et al. Association between early nutrition support and 28-day mortality in critically ill patients: the FRANS prospective nutrition cohort study. Crit Care. 2023;27(1):7.
44. Reignier J, Plantefeve G, Mira JP, Argaud L, Asfar P, Aissaoui N, et al. Low versus standard calorie and protein feeding in ventilated adults with shock: a randomized, controlled, multicentre, open-label, parallel-group trial (NUTRIREA-3). Lancet Respir Med. 2023;11(7):602–12. S2213-2600(23)00092-9.
45. Oshima T, Deutz NE, Doig G, Wischmeyer PE, Pichard C. Protein-energy nutrition in the ICU is the power couple: a hypothesis forming analysis. Clin Nutr. 2016;35(4):968–74.
46. Reid CL. Poor agreement between continuous measurements of energy expenditure and routinely used prediction equations in intensive care unit patients. Clin Nutr. 2007;26(5):649–57.
47. Alberda C, Gramlich L, Jones N, Jeejeebhoy K, Day AG, Dhaliwal R, et al. The relationship between nutritional intake and clinical outcomes in critically ill patients: results of an international multicenter observational study. Intensive Care Med. 2009;35(10):1728–37.
48. Heyland DK, Murch L, Cahill N, McCall M, Muscedere J, Stelfox HT, et al. Enhanced protein-energy provision via the enteral route feeding protocol in critically ill patients: results of a cluster randomized trial. Crit Care Med. 2013;41(12):2743–53.
49. Tsai J-R, Change W-T, Sheu C-C, Wu Y-J, Sheu Y-H, Liu P-L, et al. Inadequate energy delivery during early critical illness correlates with increased risk of mortality in patients who survive at least seven days: a retrospective study. Clin Nutr. 2011;30:209–14.
50. Ishibashi N, Plank LD, Sando K, Hill GL. Optimal protein requirements during the first 2 weeks after the onset of critical illness. Crit Care Med. 1998;26(9):1529–35.
51. Zusman O, Theilla M, Cohen J, Kagan I, Bendavid I, Singer P. Resting energy expenditure, calorie and protein consumption in critically ill patients: a retrospective cohort study. Crit Care. 2016;20(1):367.
52. Lee ZY, Yap CSL, Hasan MS, Engkasan JP, Barakatun-Nisak MY, Day AG, et al. The effect of higher versus lower protein delivery in critically ill patients: a systematic review and meta-analysis of randomized controlled trials. Crit Care. 2021;25(1):260.
53. Heyland DK, Patel J, Compher C, Rice TW, Bear DE, Lee ZY, et al. The effect of higher protein dosing in critically ill patients with high nutritional risk (EFFORT Protein): an international, multicentre, pragmatic, registry-based randomised trial. Lancet. 2023;401(10376):568–76.
54. Koekkoek W, van Setten CHC, Olthof LE, Kars J, van Zanten ARH. Timing of PROTein INtake and clinical outcomes of adult critically ill patients on prolonged mechanical VENTilation: the PROTINVENT retrospective study. Clin Nutr. 2019;38(2):883–90.
55. Cermak NM, Res PT, de Groot LC, Saris WH, van Loon LJ. Protein supplementation augments the adaptive response of skeletal muscle to resistance-type exercise training: a meta-analysis. Am J Clin Nutr. 2012;96(6):1454–64.
56. Parry SM, Knight LD, Connolly B, Baldwin C, Puthucheary Z, Morris P, et al. Factors influencing physical activity and rehabilitation in survivors of critical illness: a systematic review of quantitative and qualitative studies. Intensive Care Med. 2017;43(4):531–42.
57. Bear DE, Langan A, Dimidi D, Wandrag L, Harridge SDR, Hart N, et al. β-hydroxy-β-methylbutyrate and its impact on skeletal muscle mass and physical function in clinical practice: a systematic review and meta-analysis. Am J Clin Nutr. 2019;109(4):1119–32.
58. Viana M, Becce F, Pantet O, Schmidt S, Bagnoud G, Thaden J, et al. Impact of β-hydroxy-β-methylbutyrate (HMB) on muscle loss and protein metabolism in critically ill patients: a RCT. Clin Nutr. 2021;40:4878–87.
59. Nakamura K, Kihata A, Naraba H, Kanda N, Takahashi Y, Sonoo T, et al. β-hydroxy-β-methylbutyrate, arginine, and glutamine complex on muscle volume loss in critically ill patients: a randomized control trial. JPEN J Parenter Enteral Nutr. 2020;44(2):205–12.
60. Bear DE, Puthucheary ZA. Designing nutrition-based interventional trials for the future: addressing the known knowns. Crit Care. 2019;23(1):53.

61. Molinger J, Pastva AM, Whittle J, Wischmeyer PE. Novel approaches to metabolic assessment and structured exercise to promote recovery in ICU survivors. Curr Opin Crit Care. 2020;26(4):369–78.
62. Peterson SJ, Tsai AA, Scala CM, Sowa DC, Sheean PM, Braunschweig CL. Adequacy of oral intake in critically ill patients 1 week after extubation. J Am Diet Assoc. 2010;110(3):427–33.
63. Ridley EJ, Parke RL, Davies AR, Bailey M, Hodgson C, Deane AM, et al. What happens to nutrition intake in the post-intensive care unit hospitalization period? An observational cohort study in critically ill adults. JPEN J Parenter Enteral Nutr. 2019;43(1):88–95.
64. Wittholz K, Fetterplace K, Clode M, George ES, MacIsaac CM, Judson R, et al. Measuring nutrition-related outcomes in a cohort of multi-trauma patients following intensive care unit discharge. J Hum Nutr Diet. 2020;33:414–22.
65. Moisey LL, Pikul J, Keller H, Yeung CYE, Rahman A, Heyland DK, et al. Adequacy of protein and energy intake in critically ill adults following liberation from mechanical ventilation is dependent on route of nutrition delivery. Nutr Clin Pract. 2020;36:201–11.
66. Merriweather JL, Salisbury LG, Walsh TS, Smith P. Nutritional care after critical illness: a qualitative study of patients' experiences. J Hum Nutr Diet. 2016;29(2):127–36.
67. Merriweather J, Smith P, Walsh T. Nutritional rehabilitation after ICU—does it happen: a qualitative interview and observational study. J Clin Nurs. 2014;23(5–6):654–62.
68. van Zanten ARH, De Waele E, Wischmeyer PE. Nutrition therapy and critical illness: practical guidance for the ICU, post-ICU, and long-term convalescence phases. Crit Care. 2019;23(1):368.
69. Manley K, Hills V, Marriot S. Person-centred care: principle of nursing practice D. Nurs Stand. 2011;25:35–7.
70. Williams CM. The identification of family members' contribution to patients' care in the intensive care unit: a naturalistic inquiry. Nurs Crit Care. 2005;10(1):6–14.

Promoting Independence

5

Camilla Dawson

5.1   Introduction: What Is Dysphagia?

Dysphagia is a disruption or disorder of the total process of eating and drinking which can happen at any stage from the point food or fluid enters the oral cavity to when it leaves the oesophagus [1]. When an individual experiences disordered swallowing, food or fluid may pass into the larynx, to the level of the vocal cords (penetration) or below the level of the vocal cords (aspiration) (see Figs. 5.1 and 5.2 for pictures of a larynx in a healthy and disordered swallow). This usually causes an individual to cough or choke, their oxygen levels may drop, and they may later develop chest infections and other complications such as dehydration and malnutrition.

Patients who aspirate are 11 times more likely to develop pneumonia than those who do not aspirate [2]. Aspiration and dysphagia are different; whilst they frequently co-exist, dysphagia can be present without aspiration. When people experience 'silent aspiration', food or fluid passes into the larynx, past the vocal cords and into the trachea and or lungs without any of the symptoms mentioned previously. Patients who silently aspirate are particularly challenging to manage as they may only demonstrate late symptoms of aspiration such as chest infections which are prevalent in many patients within the ICU setting with or without dysphagia; thus, the timely, sensitive and specific differential diagnosis of dysphagia and aspiration is paramount.

5tag
C. Dawson (✉)
Queen Elizabeth Hospital, Birmingham, UK
e-mail: Camilla.dawson@nhs.net

© The Author(s), under exclusive license to Springer Nature Switzerland AG 2024
C. Boulanger, D. McWilliams (eds.), *Passport to Successful Outcomes for Patients Admitted to ICU*, https://doi.org/10.1007/978-3-031-53019-7_5

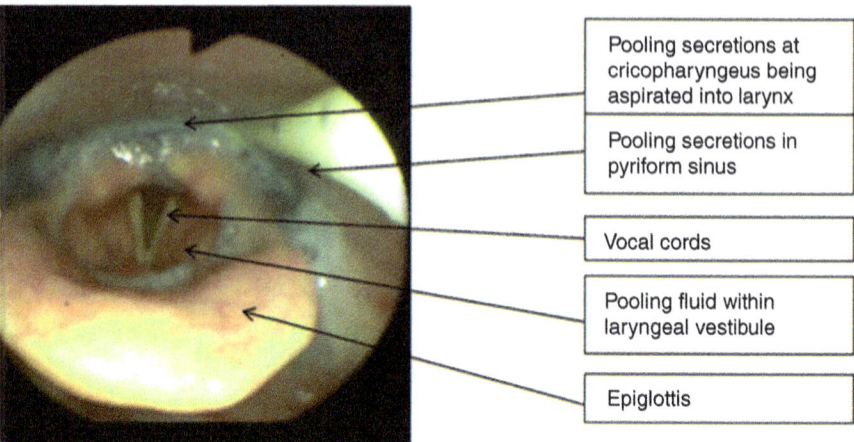

	Pooling secretions at cricopharyngeus being aspirated into larynx
	Pooling secretions in pyriform sinus
	Vocal cords
	Pooling fluid within laryngeal vestibule
	Epiglottis

Fig. 5.1 Healthy larynx

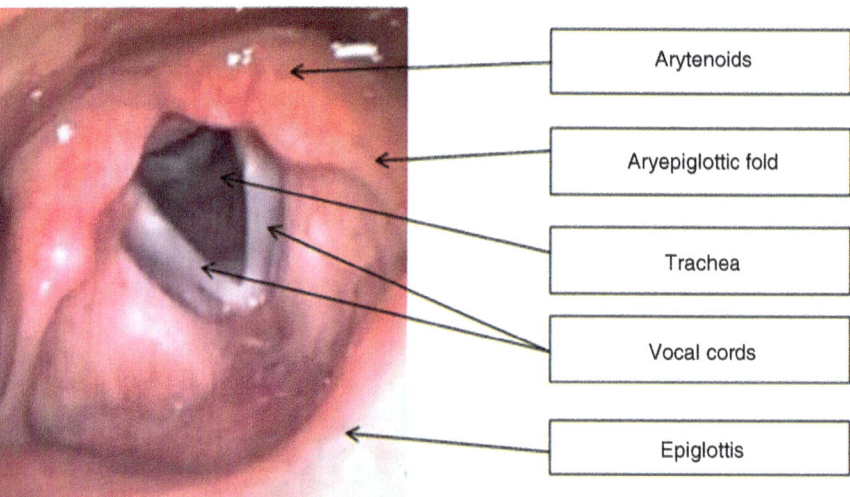

Arytenoids
Aryepiglottic fold
Trachea
Vocal cords
Epiglottis

Fig. 5.2 Disordered swallow

5.2   Dysphagia Assessment and Screening

There are numerous ways dysphagia may be assessed, from bedside screening to formal objective assessment by the speech and language therapist (SLT). Informal screening may be carried out by the multi-disciplinary team (MDT) at the bedside, monitoring for signs of dysphagia such as coughing or choking or patients reporting problems or pain on swallow [3]. Similarly, team members may notice food debris in secretions when suctioning from a tracheostomy, suggesting that food and drink is passing below the level of the vocal cords and into the trachea. These clinical symptoms should raise suspicion of dysphagia or aspiration and should trigger a referral to the SLT, allowing a formal assessment of swallowing to be carried out. Within the UK National Health Service, the SLT leads the assessment, diagnosis and management of dysphagia [1].

Many institution and condition-specific tools have been developed to support screening for dysphagia in the ICU [4, 5]. Important confounding variables impact on the usability of these screening tools, including their poor sensitivity and specificity [6] and issues such as silent aspiration, which by its very nature cannot be identified in bedside examinations. When silent aspiration may be prevalent in up to 25% of patients [7, 8], it is unlikely that screening tools alone are sufficient to identify dysphagia or aspiration. We suggest and subscribe to regular skills and awareness training from the SLT to the multi-disciplinary team in the ICU, as an effective way to educate and support clinicians to recognise symptoms and risk factors and to refer to SLT in a prompt way.

Beyond screening, many other tools are available to measure the degree of dysphagia a person presents with (see Zuercher et al. [9]); however, these are rarely standardised on patients who have dysphagia in the ICU. It is important to remember that this patient group, the care they receive, and the environment of the ICU is a complex conglomerate; non-specific tools may not capture some of these fundamental and core issues. Notwithstanding this limitation, these tools have clinical value as they enable the clinician and patient to describe the severity of the presenting dysphagia and to denote change. Patient-reported outcome measures can also be beneficial in the ICU [10], providing specific information to the clinician about the patient's experience, priorities and aims of treatment, whilst empowering and supporting the individual to become an equal partner in rehabilitation, encouraging them to recover independence.

5.3 Bedside Assessment

Formal assessment from the SLT may include bedside observation of swallow, where the SLT will provide the patient with a variety and complexity hierarchy of foods and drinks to swallow. The SLT will carefully assess and progress swallow trials, monitoring for signs of dysphagia and aspiration. As swallow issues become apparent, the SLT can implement strategies such as postural adaptations, exercises and in some cases augmentation to either the consistency or viscosity of food and drink, supporting swallow safety and efficiency. Within health care systems limited by resources including time and funding, this bedside approach to swallow management is pragmatic and effective. However, recognising the prevalence of silent aspiration and complex aetiologies in this cohort of patients, the role and value of instrumentation in swallow assessment and management are fundamental and cannot be overlooked.

5.4   Instrumental Assessment of Swallow

Instrumental assessment can include Fiberoptic Endoscopic Evaluation of Swallow (FEES) or Videofluoroscopy (VF). A FEES examination involves passing a nasendoscope through the nasopharynx and watching the larynx and pharynx during swallow (as in Figs. 5.1 and 5.2), monitoring for aspiration and assessing the degree of dysphagia. This also provides an ideal opportunity for the SLT to provide rehabilitation strategies or compensation support as required, monitoring in real time for aspiration. This laryngeal evaluation also enables examination of vocal fold movement and laryngeal/pharyngeal sensation and can be completed on the ward. Conversely, VF is completed in the radiology department, it is a moving X-ray of a person swallowing various radiopaque consistencies of diet and fluids. This assessment provides a unique perspective, enabling the SLT to view the oropharynx, larynx and upper oesophagus simultaneously. The biofeedback provided to the patient who is able to visualise their own swallow is also of great value. Challenges of VF include the ability to move patients who are ventilated or who are difficult to position within the fluoroscopy suite; however, this is institution specific. Benefits and challenges of VF and FEES have been debated, and each yields significant improvement to the assessment and management of people with dysphagia and the MDT supporting them [11, 12].

Once the SLT has assessed swallow, recommendations regarding fluid and diet consistencies will be made. It is important to use clear obvious language to describe swallow recommendations, avoiding ambiguity or interpretation by the wider team. The International Dysphagia Diet Standards (IDDSI) is a standardised approach to describe the consistency of food and fluids and should be employed by SLT teams.

5.5   Causes and Presentations of Dysphagia in the ICU

Dysphagia may occur as a result of numerous etiologies including but not limited to trauma, head and neck cancer, spinal cord injury, neurological issues, cardiovascular surgery, respiratory issues and intubation [9]. The efferent and afferent sensory motor pathways from the brain stem to the upper airway and oesophagus co-ordinate and facilitate safe and effective swallowing. When these pathways or the anatomy around them are disrupted, the individual may experience dysphagia. Patients frequently present with multiple causes of their dysphagia grounded in physiological issues such as global weakness and critical care neuropathies alongside anatomical issues such as a dislocated arytenoid due to intubation injury, or neck trauma impacting on pharyngeal competence for example. It is important that the diagnosis of dysphagia is achieved in a comprehensive way, to include the likely mechanism of injury, with a clear description of the nature of dysphagia and or aspiration, suggested therapeutic and rehabilitative interventions and hypothesised treatment trajectory. Whilst it can be challenging to define these criteria and treatment plans when so many concurrent clinical issues exist, it is important that dysphagia is recognised and described in a logical, comprehensive and scientific way.

The MDT and SLT need to be mindful of the fluctuant swallow and the non-linearity in swallow competence for patients in the ICU. Unlike other circumstances where dysphagia may exist and be rehabilitated and managed in a somewhat predictable way, swallow competence within the ICU may not progress in an expected or incremental way. With concurrent presentations such as critical care neuropathies, sarcopenia, increased gastro-oesophageal reflux, Acute Respiratory Distress Syndrome (ARDS), altered consciousness and delirium and the use of sedatives [3], the dysphagia presentation may also fluctuate and change as a result of alterations to any of these variables. Muscle weakness, fatigue, sensation changes in the pharynx and larynx, breathe–swallow coordination challenge and reduced cognitive awareness associated with eating and drinking all contribute to an individual's swallowing problems. These issues need to be regularly and comprehensively assessed to manage dysphagia in a proactive rather than a reactive way.

5.6 Post-extubation Dysphagia

Intubation involves the placement of an endotracheal tube through the pharynx and larynx to support mechanical ventilation. The placement of this tube can cause iatrogenic injury to the larynx and pharynx such as damage to the mucosa, along with physiological alterations to sensation [13, 14]; however, other dysphagia risk factors may also relate to the individual's primary diagnosis. Post-extubation dysphagia is an important issue as it is significantly associated with aspiration pneumonia, reintubation, increased length of stay and surgical placement of feeding tubes [15].

The frequency of dysphagia following endotracheal intubation ranges from 3% to 62% across diagnostic subtypes and is related to the duration of intubation, with longer periods of intubation associated with a higher incidence of post-extubation dysphagia [16]. These findings have also been reflected in patient's self-reporting dysphagia at the point of discharge from ICU, identifying a relationship between the duration of intubation and perceived dysphagia [17]. Recent research has identified a statistically significant relationship between the laryngeal adductor reflex, aspiration and duration of intubation [18]. This important information may enable teams to begin to stratify patients who are at greater risk of aspiration due to the duration of intubation, creating personalised protocols and assessments.

Timely and accurate assessment of dysphagia is important for this cohort of patients, utilising both bedside assessment and objective measures such as FEES and VF; however, identifying what therapeutic interventions may be appropriate can be challenging. There are limited research studies which explore what interventions are optimal for specific dysphagia presentations, and there are no research studies which define what treatment regimens are optimal for this cohort of patients. Additionally, there are no studies which define how often or frequently swallow exercises should be carried out to optimise outcomes in this cohort of patients. Instead, Speech and Language Therapists need a robust understanding of the principles of rehabilitation, along with high level clinical and perceptual ability to continually assess diagnose and manage dysphagia, adapting to alterations in the clinical presentation of patients in the ICU.

5.7   Ventilation and Dysphagia

Breathing and swallowing are highly coordinated, complex processes, utilising many of the same muscle groups, moderated by neural control centres in the dorso-medial and ventrolateral medulla [19]. The coordination and synchronisation of these processes are critical to consider when assessing and managing dysphagia. As an overview, the pattern of breathing and swallowing involves closure of the glottis, the opening of the cricopharyngeus and the descent of bolus through the oropharynx and upper oesophagus before breathing recommences. When patients have a brief apnoeic phase as the vocal cords adduct, the transit of bolus through the upper aerodigestive tract can be compromised, the glottis can remain open or partially open as bolus passes through it and opening of the cricopharyngeus may be miss-timed, resulting in penetration and or aspiration. These particular issues are pertinent when patients are or have been receiving mechanical ventilation.

When patients require oxygen supplementation and respiratory support, the natural respiratory rate may alter, challenging the automatic regulation of the breathe–swallow interaction. Experience suggests that it can be particularly challenging for patients who are globally decompensated to manage their breathe–swallow coordination when positive pressure is being delivered via a tracheostomy with a cuff inflated or deflated. In this circumstance, the apposition of the vocal cords can be disrupted and any leak airflow can have a negative impact on swallow timing which can be difficult to improve during the respiratory wean. Interventions and adaptations to ventilation settings can, however, be made to help improve the control and success of communication. Research has identified that when lengthened inspiratory time and positive end expiratory pressure (PEEP) changes are made to the ventilator, patients can achieve greater duration of phonation time, with greater volume, articulation and quality of speech [20].

The respiratory wean and liberation form ventilator support is a critical time for patients with dysphagia in ICU. As the patient begins to work harder to breathe independently, their reliance on ventilation and potential transition through spontaneous breathing trials, to pressure support and or continuous positive airway pressure (CPAP) is an important variable to account for. This is especially pertinent for the patient that may be swallowing oral intake and being ventilated via a tracheostomy.

As the respiratory wean progresses and the patient gradually regains strength and independence, fatigue and increased respiratory effort are important to note. To manage dysphagia effectively, it is important to recognise subtle changes in ventilator settings which require proactive dysphagia management. For example, if a patient needs increasing durations of 'rest' on pressure support, it may be pertinent to cease oral intake during this rest, as the patient fatigues, to reduce the risk of aspiration-related compromise. Conversely, to improve strength and tolerance of the respiratory wean, facilitating leak speech and speaking valve trials to improve laryngeal sensation and competence can be of benefit. Proactively optimising nutrition and hydration via alternative means such as naso-gastric feeding during times of fluctuant or low oral intake is vital. Little nutritional benefit will be achieved if the patient swallows small volumes, inconsistently, when fatigued-risking malnutrition, dehydration and aspiration.

It is also important to note the potential impact of high flow oxygen via nasal cannula on swallow competence. This is a relatively new approach to oxygen delivery and in the absence of large randomised controlled trials, small case series which demonstrate experience of dysphagia in this cohort are of great value. A recent study identified decreased swallow function in healthy subjects who had swallow assessment when receiving high-flow nasal cannula flow rate of >40 L/min [21], reiterating the importance of timely and where possible, instrumental assessment of swallow.

5.8   Tracheostomy and Dysphagia

The impact of tracheostomy on swallow is a complex topic. Over the past 40 years, publications have either wholly endorsed a significant relationship between tracheostomy and dysphagia [22] or refuted any such relationship [23]. A recent scoping review has established a significant risk of bias in the available research with regard to dysphagia assessment consistency, operational definitions and blinding [24]. This information is important, as it orientates the clinician to the limitations of available evidence and, therefore, the importance of avoiding reductionist or binary statements about whether a tracheostomy either does or does not impact on swallow competence. It is pragmatic to recognise that when a tracheostomy coexists with dysphagia it may exacerbate and contribute to symptoms a person presents with-especially when the cuff is inflated [25]. Each patient with a tracheostomy requires careful individual assessment and management, considering alterations and adaptations to the tracheostomy where appropriate such as fenestrating the tube, reducing the lumen of the tube or using a speaking valve.

There are a range of different types of tracheostomies and speaking valves. These include those with adjustable flanges, cuffed or uncuffed, made out of soft silicone, plastic or silver, and with or without fenestration. To promote independence, early facilitation of voice, communication and swallow is paramount. The ability to adapt and change the tracheostomy, modify the lumen of airflow through and around the tracheostomy, and use of one way speaking valves should not be overlooked by the team, as subtle changes can support improved function. The passey-muir valve can also be of benefit to patients who are ventilated, to support the restoration of airflow through the pharynx and to improve tidal volumes [26].

5.8.1 COVID-19

SARS-CoV-2 had a complex and multi system impact on individuals who contracted the virus and required intensive care support. From a dysphagia and upper airway perspective, many patients have presented with unique clinical issues, different to other cohorts of patients with respiratory compromise. Empirical data has identified important features, specifically upper airway oedema, impaired airway protection and aspiration which has been associated with longer total artificial airway duration, longer tracheostomy tube duration, multiple intubations and was associated with persistent ICU acquired weakness at ICU discharge [27]. Careful examination and assessment of the upper airway and potential mechanism of injury to the whole process of breathing and swallowing is required for this group of patients. Evidence suggests that the synchronicity of breathing and swallowing can become fundamentally compromised for people who are critically ill with COVID-19, where these systems are in competition rather than working alongside one another [27].

It is important to note that studies exploring acute dysphagia and COVID-19 frequently reported swallow function returning to pre morbid function at the point of discharge from hospital [28, 29]; however the prevalence of ongoing self-reported voice and swallow problems up to a year post ICU discharge has been reported in 34% and 20% respectively [30]. This large prospective study found that 60% with swallow problems received invasive mechanical ventilation and were more likely to have undergone proning. Voice problems were reported in 34% post-ICU admission and these patients were more likely to have received invasive or non-invasive ventilation and to have been proned. These conglomerate issues are important to note, supporting clinicians to identify which patients may be at greatest risk of swallowing problems; those who are proned and receive mechanical ventilation, and people with tracheostomies with upper airway oedema and compromised airway protection. The total rehabilitation journey is inextricably linked to swallow and upper airway function in people who are critically ill with COVID-19. Clinical teams require proactive, agile and skilled services to identify, assess and manage swallow disorders, reducing the burden and sequalae of aspiration events and their impact.

5.9   Rehabilitation Principles

Specific institutions employ various approaches to commencing oral intake, whilst a patient is ventilated via a tracheostomy. A patient-centred approach is key and there are no absolute rules regarding the point at which patients may commence oral intake, rather this decision is based on the clinical presentation of the patient. As a minimum, automatic triggers for SLT referral should be considered before commencing swallow trials for patients who have:

- The cuff inflated and are receiving ventilation via tracheostomy.
- Patients who are on flat bed rest due to spinal cord injury and ventilated.

- Patients who have had a prolonged period of intubation >72 h.
- Those who have multiple failed extubations.
- Patients who are ventilated following lung transplantation and are due to be extubated.

It is our experience that those with the aforementioned presentations are at great risk of silent aspiration so require a timely instrumental assessment of swallow from the SLT in the first instance. This list is not exhaustive.

Swallow rehabilitation is an important facet of regaining and promoting independence after care in the ICU. Whilst much of this chapter has orientated the reader to the medicalisation of swallow and the physiological effects of dysphagia, the social meaning of eating and drinking should always be recognised by clinicians. Anthropological studies define the social, religious and cultural processes associated with eating and drinking [31]. In 'The Anthropology of Food and Eating', Mintz and Du Bois [31] explain that *"Next to breathing, eating is perhaps the most essential of all human activities, and one with which much of social life is entwined"* (p. 102). The rituals associated with eating and drinking are fundamental when considering how we may promote independence. To enable someone to capably eat and drink can support the liberation from ventilation, feeding tubes and reliance on nutritional supplements. Returning to normal meals and eating routine can also support sleep–wake cycles and a sense of well-being.

5.10 Swallow Rehabilitation

Following the careful and instrumental assessment of swallow, management options are grounded in either providing compensation strategies or specific exercise-based rehabilitation to improve strength, coordination and overall function [32, 33]. There are no studies which have identified specific swallow rehabilitation programmes or protocols for patients in ICU owing to the heterogeneous cohort and multiple causes of dysphagia.

In the first instance, least restrictive measures should be put in place to improve swallow competence, enabling the individual to engage with qualitative benefits of eating and drinking, whilst protecting what may be precarious chest status exacerbated by dysphagia. This may include manoeuvres such as a head turn towards the side of a vocal cord palsy or pharyngeal weakness, to preclude food or fluid passing through structures unable to provide sufficient motor function to control flow and passage of bolus. Early injection laryngoplasty for patients with vocal cord palsy can also be of great value for patients in the ICU, promoting quality voice use and improving swallow competence [34]. Using a chin tuck posture also has the potential to improve swallow function, opening the vallecula and slowing down bolus flow for patients who may experience pre- or intra-swallow aspiration.

Exercises to improve swallow competence include strengthening the tongue base by placing the tongue between the teeth (Masako) and swallowing. The 'supraglottic swallow' encourages the individual to close the vocal cords pre-swallow, to help protect the laryngeal inlet from penetration or aspiration. The 'super-supraglottic swallow' involves a cough release post-swallow, to proactively expectorate any aspirated material. The 'Mendelsohn manoeuver' works on squeezing pharyngeal musculature to improve tension and tone.

In rare circumstances, the use of thickening agents may be used as a rehabilitation tool to enable specific patients to commence oral intake. This may be helpful for patients with oral control issues, or when FEES or VF demonstrates the benefit of thickened fluids. For patients who have a spinal injury, or trauma resulting in flat bed rest, McRae [35] explains the limitations of pharyngeal contraction during swallow due to potential compromise to ansa cervicalis, coupled with poor positioning, phrenic nerve dysfunction and loss of the cough reflex. These concurrent issues alert the clinician to the potential risk associated with swallowing thickened fluids, sticky and challenging to remove from the pharynx and even more challenging to expectorate from the lungs. This type of patient-specific data should always drive the choice and management of swallow rehabilitation plans.

When patients have issues with mastication fatigue or positioning, diet modification such as choosing softer or blended foods may be of benefit for a discreet period as the patient regains function. It is our experience that swallow rehabilitation may be optimised when volume, consistency of fluid and diet are all carefully considered and administered, alongside targeted exercise regimes to improve swallow competence. FEES and VF are fundamental to guide these interventions and to help engage and encourage the patient to adhere to what may be frustrating and limiting therapeutic plans-albeit with the aim of regaining independence. There are no published exercise regimes or suggested frequency or intensity of exercise rehabilitation for swallow therapy in the ICU. As the discipline develops and the available literature expands to include these details, therapists are encouraged to use robust theoretical underpinning and justification for their interventions. With a patient cohort who has a high propensity for dysphagia, it is equally insufficient to blindly prescribe normal diet and fluids, thickened fluids, nil by mouth status or alternative means of feeding without careful and considered assessment and risk management.

5.11 Conclusion

The ICU is a unique clinical environment, supporting the most vulnerable patients. To promote independence and optimise function, it is important that the multidisciplinary team works together to recognise, identify and effectively manage swallow compromise. The collective skills of the Speech and Language Therapist, Ear Nose and Throat Surgeons, Physiotherapist, Intensivist, Dietitian and Occupational Therapist are fundamental to promote independence and improve function. Interventions to improve swallow should be guided by comprehensive assessment, along with the holistic context and well-being of the individual, developing and changing in an iterative way as the individual's status improves or deteriorates. Swallowing simultaneously exists within sociological and medical paradigms. Overlooking either one of these components underestimates the complexity and importance of dysphagia therapy to metaphorically and physically nourish the individual and promote independence and successful discharge.

Key Take Home Messages

- There is high prevalence of dysphagia and aspiration in patients within ICU, consider these issues in differential diagnosis, especially when aspiration may be silent.
- Swallow competence is intimately related to breathing, think about swallow competence when patients are undergoing respiratory weaning.
- Rehabilitation and recovery of swallow competence may be non-linear, swallow may not recover as quickly as mobility, remember this at important milestones such as liberation from the ventilator and tracheostomy decannulation.
- We need to assess, manage and provide swallow therapy with robust, clear rationale and evidence, not overlooking the science of swallow rehabilitation and the fundamental role of the SLT to lead this intervention.

References

1. RCSLT. In: Taylor-Goh S, editor. Royal College of Speech & Language Therapists clinical guidelines. 3rd ed. Speechmark: Bicestor; 2005.
2. Martino R, Foley N, Bhogal S, Diamant N, Speechley M, Teasell R. Dysphagia after stroke: incidence, diagnosis, and pulmonary complications. Stroke. 2005;36(12):2756–63.
3. Schefold JC, Berger D, Zurcher P, Lensch M, Perren A, Jakob SM, et al. Dysphagia in mechanically ventilated ICU patients (DYnAMICS): a prospective observational trial. Crit Care Med. 2017;45(12):2061–9.
4. Warner HL, Suiter DM, Nystrom KV, Poskus K, Leder SB. Comparing accuracy of the Yale swallow protocol when administered by registered nurses and speech-language pathologists. J Clin Nurs. 2014;23(13–14):1908–15.
5. Leder SB, Suiter DM, Warner HL, Acton I M, Swainson BA. Success of recommending oral diets in acute stroke patients based on passing a 90-cc water swallow challenge protocol. Top Stroke Rehabil. 2012;19(1):40–4.
6. Johnson KL, Speirs L, Mitchell A, Przybyl H, Anderson D, Manos B, et al. Validation of a postextubation dysphagia screening tool for patients after prolonged endotracheal intubation. Am J Crit Care. 2018;27(2):89–96.
7. Ajemian MS, Nirmul GB, Anderson MT, Zirlen DM, Kwasnik EM. Routine fiberoptic endoscopic evaluation of swallowing following prolonged intubation: implications for management. Arch Surg. 2001;136(4):434–7.
8. Leder SB, Cohn SM, Moller BA. Fiberoptic endoscopic documentation of the high incidence of aspiration following extubation in critically ill trauma patients. Dysphagia. 1998;13(4):208–12.
9. Zuercher P, Moret CS, Dziewas R, Schefold JC. Dysphagia in the intensive care unit: epidemiology, mechanisms, and clinical management. Crit Care. 2019;23(1):103.
10. Patel DA, Sharda R, Hovis K, Nichols E, Sathe N, Penson D, et al. Patient-reported outcome measures in dysphagia: a systematic review of instrument development and validation. Dis Esophagus. 2017;30:1–23.
11. Langmore SE, Schatz K, Olson N. Endoscopic and videofluoroscopic evaluations of swallowing and aspiration. Ann Otol Rhinol Laryngol. 1991;100(8):678–81.

12. Kelly AM, Drinnan MJ, Leslie P. Assessing penetration and aspiration: how do video-fluoroscopy and fiberoptic endoscopic evaluation of swallowing compare? Laryngoscope. 2007;117(10):1723–7.
13. Brodsky MB, Gonzalez-Fernandez M, Mendez-Tellez PA, Shanholtz C, Palmer JB, Needham DM. Factors associated with swallowing assessment after oral endotracheal intubation and mechanical ventilation for acute lung injury. Ann Am Thorac Soc. 2014;11(10):1545–52.
14. Macht M, Wimbish T, Clark BJ, Benson AB, Burnham EL, Williams A, et al. Diagnosis and treatment of post-extubation dysphagia: results from a national survey. J Crit Care. 2012;27(6):578–86.
15. Macht M, Wimbish T, Clark BJ, Benson AB, Burnham EL, Williams A, et al. Postextubation dysphagia is persistent and associated with poor outcomes in survivors of critical illness. Crit Care. 2011;15(5):R231.
16. Skoretz S, Flowers H, Martino R. The incidence of dysphagia following endotracheal intubation a systematic review. Chest. 2010;137:665–73.
17. Brodsky MB, Gellar JE, Dinglas VD, Colantuoni E, Mendez-Tellez PA, Shanholtz C, et al. Duration of oral endotracheal intubation is associated with dysphagia symptoms in acute lung injury patients. J Crit Care. 2014;29(4):574–9.
18. Borders JC, Fink D, Levitt JE, McKeehan J, McNally E, Rubio A, et al. Relationship between laryngeal sensation, length of intubation, and aspiration in patients with acute respiratory failure. Dysphagia. 2019;34(4):521–8.
19. Martin-Harris B. Coordination of respiration and swallowing. GI Motility Online; 2006.
20. Hoit JD, Banzett RB, Lohmeier HL, Hixon TJ, Brown R. Clinical ventilator adjustments that improve speech. Chest. 2003;124(4):1512–21.
21. Oomagari M, Fujishima I, Katagiri N, Arizono S, Watanabe K, Ohno T, et al. Swallowing function during high-flow nasal cannula therapy. Eur Respir J. 2015;46(Suppl 59):PA4199.
22. Bonanno P. Swallowing dysfunction after tracheostomy. Ann Surg. 1971;174(1):29.
23. Leder SB, Ross DA. Confirmation of no causal relationship between tracheotomy and aspiration status: a direct replication study. Dysphagia. 2010;25(1):35–9.
24. Skoretz SA, Riopelle S, Wellman L, Dawson C. Investigating swallowing and tracheostomy following critical illness: a scoping review. Crit Care Med. 2019;48:e141. https://doi.org/10.1097/CCM.0000000000004098.
25. Amathieu R, Sauvat S, Reynaud P, Slavov V, Luis D, Dinca A, et al. Influence of the cuff pressure on the swallowing reflex in tracheostomized intensive care unit patients. Br J Anaesth. 2012;109(4):578–83.
26. Sutt A-L, Caruana LR, Dunster KR, Cornwell PL, Anstey CM, Fraser JF. Speaking valves in tracheostomised ICU patients weaning off mechanical ventilation—do they facilitate lung recruitment? Crit Care. 2016;20(1):91.
27. Dawson C, Nankivell P, Pracy JP, et al. Functional laryngeal assessment in patients with tracheostomy following COVID-19 a prospective cohort study. Dysphagia. 2023;38(2):657–66.
28. Dawson C, Capewell R, Ellis S, Matthews S, Adamson S, Wood M, et al. Dysphagia presentation and management following coronavirus disease 2019: an acute care tertiary centre experience. J Laryngol Otol. 2020;134(11):981–6. https://doi.org/10.1017/S0022215120002443.
29. Archer SK, Iezzi CM, Gilpin L. Swallowing and voice outcomes in patients hospitalized with COVID-19: an observational cohort study. Arch Phys Med Rehabil. 2021;102(6):1084–90. https://doi.org/10.1016/j.apmr.2021.01.063. Epub 2021 Jan 30. PMID: 33529610; PMCID: PMC7846878.
30. Dawson C, Clunie G, Evison F, et al. Prevalence of swallow, communication, voice and cognitive compromise following hospitalisation for COVID-19: the PHOSP-COVID analysis. BMJ Open Respir Res. 2023;10:e001647. https://doi.org/10.1136/bmjresp-2023-001647.
31. Mintz SW, Du Bois CM. The anthropology of food and eating. Annu Rev Anthropol. 2002;31:99–119.
32. The Faculty of Intensive Care Medicine, Society. AIC. Guidelines for the provision of intensive care services. Speech and Language Therapists; 2019.

33. The Royal College of Speech and Language Therapists. Position paper, speech and language therapy in adult critical care; 2014.
34. Choi N, Jin H, Kim HJ, Son YI. Early injection laryngoplasty with a long-lasting material in patients with potentially recoverable unilateral vocal fold paralysis. Clin Exp Otorhinolaryngol. 2019;12:427–32.
35. McRae J, Smith C, Beeke S, Emmanuel A. Oropharyngeal dysphagia management in cervical spinal cord injury patients: an exploratory survey of variations to care across specialised and non-specialised units. Spinal Cord Ser Cases. 2019;5(1):31.

Mobility and Function

6

David McWilliams and Owen Gustafson

6.1 Introduction: The Impact of Bed Rest

6.1.1 Skeletal Muscles

Muscle wasting occurs early and rapidly during the first week of critical illness, with losses of up to 20% seen for those in multi-organ failure [1]. The aetiology of this muscle weakness is multifactorial including sarcopenia from pre-existing comorbidities such as frailty, disuse atrophy due to bed rest [2] and ICU acquired weakness (ICUAW) [3]. ICUAW, defined as a clinically detected weakness in critically ill patients where there is no plausible aetiology other than critical illness [4], is a consequence of acute illness and may include axonal neuropathy, myopathy or both. ICUAW affects 25–100% of the critical care population with risk factors including sepsis, use of neuromuscular blocking agents, steroids, deep sedation and hyperglycaemia [5]. As well as a reduction in muscle mass, there is an associated deterioration in terms of muscle performance. Maximal knee extensor contraction (that is, maximal strength) has been shown to decrease by 22% after 14 days of bed rest [6] and as much as 53% after 28 days of limb immobilisation [7].

A strong correlation between muscular weakness and poor outcomes has been observed, with weakness directly associated with failure to wean from mechanical ventilation and increased in-hospital mortality rates [8, 9], as well as severe functional impairments and reduced pace and degree of recovery in ICU survivors

D. McWilliams (✉)
Centre for Care Excellence, Coventry University, Coventry, UK
e-mail: David.mcwilliams@uhcw.nhs.uk

O. Gustafson
Oxford Allied Health Professions Research & Innovation Unit, Oxford University Hospitals NHS Foundation Trust, John Radcliffe Hospital, Oxford, UK
e-mail: Owen.Gustafson@ouh.nhs.uk

[10]. These effects can last months to years after hospital discharge [11], with a negative impact on employment and income in ICU survivors and their caregivers, and mortality and utilisation of primary care services are high in the immediate post-discharge period [12]. This was perhaps most notably seen in the recent COVID-19 pandemic, where unprecedented numbers of patients were admitted to intensive care units with severe illness requiring prolonged periods of deep sedation and mechanical ventilation. As a consequence, rates of initial and residual ICUAW were high [13], and up to two thirds of survivors requiring ongoing community rehabilitation following hospital discharge [14].

6.1.2 Respiratory Muscles

In the presence of critical illness, there is a reduction in diaphragmatic activity, where atrophy and contractile dysfunction have been identified as early as 18 h following the onset of mechanical ventilation [15, 16]. Diaphragm dysfunction is considered to be present in up to 80% of patients with ICUAW [17]. In addition to the impact of critical illness, respiratory function is also influenced by positioning and bed rest. When in the supine position, functional residual capacity (FRC) is reduced by between 0.5 and 1 L, moving below the closing volume and causing areas of atelectasis in dependent lung regions. Clinically, this deterioration in respiratory muscles is associated with reduced cough strength and increased risk of developing ventilator-associated pneumonia [18].

6.1.3 Cardiovascular System

The cardiovascular system is also affected by a period of critical illness and immobility, demonstrating a 28% reduction in stroke volume after just 10 days of bed rest. This deterioration can lead to the development of orthostatic intolerance within just 72 h of immobility [19]. The reduction in cardiovascular fitness coupled with the reduced respiratory function already described has a subsequent effect on overall fitness, with a reduction in VO_2 max at a rate of 0.9% per day [20]. This reduced exercise capacity could contribute to delayed physical recovery, prolonged weaning from mechanical ventilation and a significantly reduced exercise capacity at the point of hospital discharge and beyond.

6.1.4 Bone

During a period of critical illness, there is also a degree of bone demineralisation as a result of a lack of weight-bearing and reduced activity levels. Bone resorption is markedly increased in critically ill patients, while markers of bone formation are decreased [21]. Specifically, studies have shown a loss of 6 mg of calcium per day from bone tissue, which equates to approximately 2% of total bone density after just

1 month of immobility [22]. This can take up to 2 years to return to the prior level of bone density, with a 20% increase in fracture risk observed in survivors of acute respiratory distress syndrome [23].

6.2   Benefits of Early Rehabilitation

The term 'early rehabilitation' within the ICU refers to interventions that commence immediately after stabilisation of physiological derangements [24]. These interventions may start within 1 or 2 days of initiation of mechanical ventilation, although often those patients most at risk of prolonged sequelae are still too acutely unwell for active mobilisation. In this instance, the focus should be placed on preventative measures such as regular positional change and passive/active exercise until mobilisation can be initiated safely. The time taken to mobilise appears to have a significant bearing on a patient's short- and long-term recovery, with increased ICU and hospital length of stay and poor functional outcomes observed in patients with delayed time to first mobilisation [25–27]. The ability to minimise the duration and subsequently the impact of critical illness associated bed rest is, therefore, of paramount importance.

Early and progressive mobilisation has been demonstrated to be both safe and feasible for patients admitted to critical care [28]. When implemented, programmes of early mobility have demonstrated numerous benefits to both the patient and the organisation. As a result, early mobilisation is now included as a key component in a number of national and international guidelines [29, 30]. At a patient level, early mobilisation helps to prevent the loss of muscle mass and minimise the poor physical condition associated with prolonged bed rest [31]. As a result, early mobilisation is associated with significant improvements in functional status, muscle strength, walking ability at discharge and health-related quality of life [32]. At an organisational level, the introduction of early mobility programmes is associated with reduced healthcare costs resulting from a reduction in ICU and hospital length of stay and subsequently improved patient flow. Early mobility has also been associated with reduced hospital readmissions, a reduction in the duration of mechanical ventilation and a reduction in both the incidence and duration of delirium [25–27].

6.3   Commencing Mobilisation

Starting mobilisation as early as clinically possible is an important method of reducing the significant impact of critical illness immobility. To help decision making, expert consensus guidelines have been produced to help decision making for the initiation of early mobilisation [33], with a systematic review and meta-analysis of over 20,000 rehabilitation interventions showing a low risk of adverse events [28]. As our knowledge and understanding of rehabilitation in ICU has increased, an increasing number of mobility protocols have been developed to support practice (see examples in Figs. 6.1 and 6.2). The use of protocols for mobilisation may have

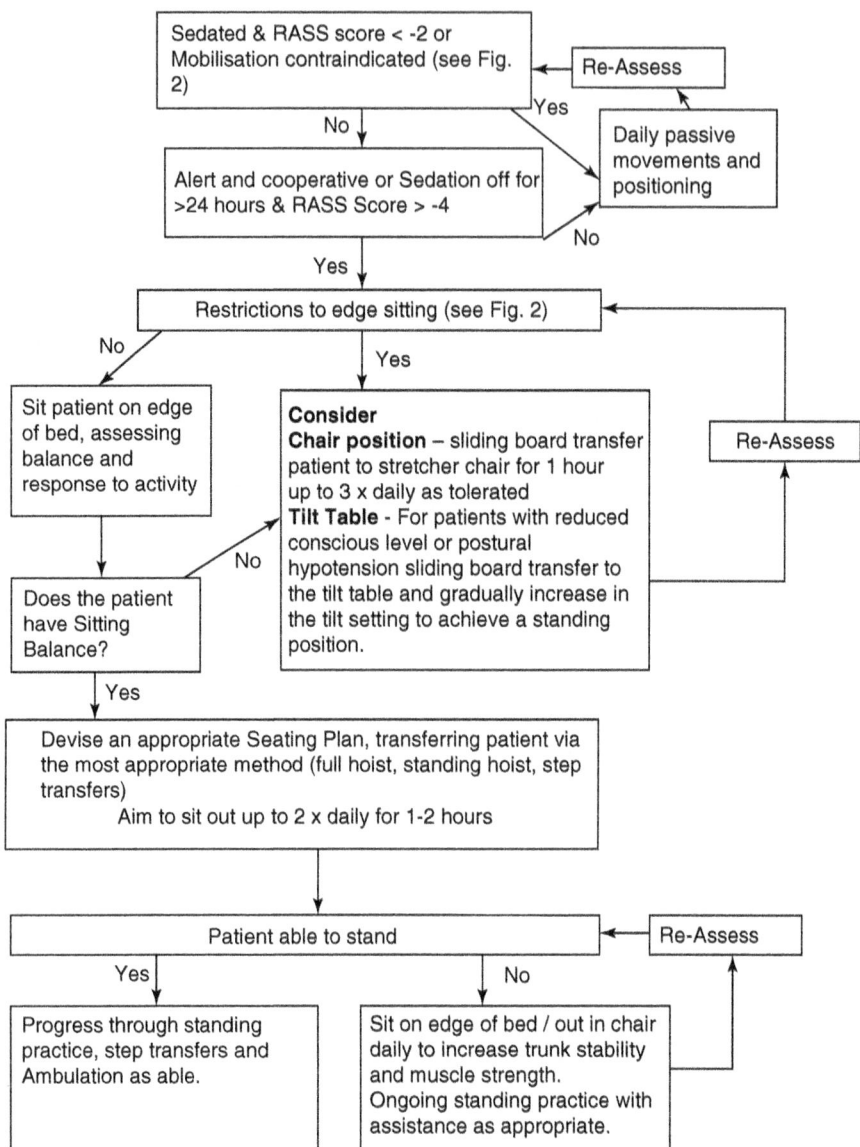

Fig. 6.1 Early and structured mobility protocol. (From McWilliams et al. [27])

a number of beneficial effects, helping to guide initiation and identify patients who are deemed sufficiently haemodynamically stable and ready to start more active mobilisation. Commencing mobilisation is, however, only the start of the rehabilitation journey and any protocol developed should also provide a structure or framework to empower healthcare professionals to progress activity and ensure ongoing collaboration between team members.

Exclusion Criteria

- Significant dose of Vasoactive agents (e.g. >0.2 mcg/kg/min noradrenaline or
  equivalent) for haemodynamic stability (Maintain Mean arterial pressure >60)
- Mechanically Ventilated with FiO2 >0.8 and/or PEEP >12 **or** acutely worsening
  respiratory failure
- Neuromuscular paralysing agent
- Acute Neurological event (e.g. CVA, SAH)
- Unstable spine or extremity fractures with contraindications to mobilise
- Active bleeding process

Restrictions to edge sitting

- Small dose of Vasoactive agents (e.g. 01 - 0.2 mcg/kg/min noradrenaline or
  equivalent) for haemodynamic stability (Maintain Mean arterial pressure >60)
- Mechanically Ventilated with FiO2 >0.6 and/or PEEP >10
- Poor tolerance of Endotracheal tube
- Open abdomen or high risk for dehiscence – liaise with surgeons prior to mobilising
- Haemofiltration via a femoral line

Fig. 6.2 Exclusion criteria and restrictions to edge sitting

Ultimately, the decision to commence mobilisation should be based on an assessment of cardiovascular stability and respiratory reserve. The arousal level should be considered, but reduced arousal is not necessarily a contraindication to rehabilitation, where supported sitting or verticalisation may serve as a stimulus to aid wakening and form part of the assessment of neurological status.

6.3.1   Sitting on Edge of the Bed

Whether the patient is ventilated or not, the process of sitting a patient on the edge of the bed forms an important part of early assessment and subsequent provision of a structured rehabilitation programme and seating plan. This process provides vital information with regard to patients' sitting balance and readiness for sitting out of bed, their physiological stability in response to activity and positional change, as well as many other specific physical and psychological benefits.

The change to an upright position challenges both the cardiovascular and respiratory systems. Following an extended stay in the ICU, patients are likely to experience the equivalent response to vigorous exercise (i.e. an increase in heart rate and respiratory rate) at even low levels of activity, such as moving from lying to sitting or completing activities of daily living such as washing. This is due to an overall reduction in the oxidative capacity of muscle [34]. This suggests that patients within critical care may benefit from the effects of training, albeit in a modified way to meet their current levels of physical capacity and reserve. Alongside the early initiation of rehabilitation, having a robust and consistent structure for rehabilitation is equally important in the proceeding days/weeks to support ongoing recovery.

To support this activity and its progression, and once sitting balance and physiological reserve have been determined, an individualised rehabilitation programme should be devised to aid recovery. In the early stages, this often involves the establishment of a seating programme. On initially sitting out of bed, critically ill patients often present with significantly limited mobility and an inability to reposition themselves independently. Coupled with nutritional deficiency, this leads to a significant increase in the risk of developing pressure ulcers [35]. To combat this, assessment should be made for the provision of specialist equipment such as wheelchairs, special seating and other postural support equipment. This may also involve the use of a high-specification foam or equivalent pressure redistributing cushion. By providing early specialist assessment and provision of pressure-relieving seating systems, the risk of developing pressure ulcers and/or contractures is reduced. Sitting out of bed regularly in this way has a number of benefits (Fig. 6.3) and is an important mainstay of treatment to support recovery.

6.3.2   Standing

Once an established seating plan has been formulated, with patients sitting out on a daily basis preferably on multiple occasions, progression can be made to more active exercise, standing and ambulation. If the patient is able to maintain their sitting balance with minimal support and move their legs against gravity, attempts can be made at standing with a number of additional benefits (Fig. 6.4). Gradually increasing muscle strength and stamina will lead to increasing levels of functional independence and have beneficial effects on a patient's psychological status as they become more independent and the improvements become more tangible. This process of mobilisation does, however, bring additional safety considerations such as

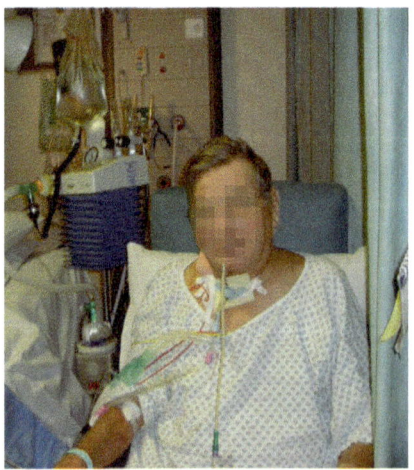

- Increased functional residual capacity

- Provides support to the trunk so less demanding from a respiratory point of view than edge sitting

- Upright posture challenges the cardiovascular system and provides orthostatic stimulus

- Provides neurological stimulus to aid waking and reorientation

- Positive psychological benefits of being out of bed

Fig. 6.3 Example of benefits of sitting out of bed

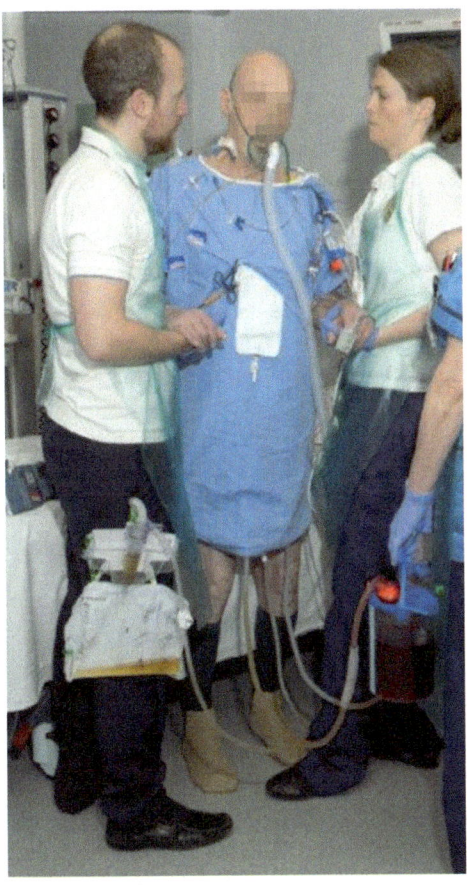

- Increased Functional residual capacity
- Increased tidal volumes
    - Weight-bearing
    - Maintain ankle range
    - Improved trunk stability
    - Postural management

Fig. 6.4 Example of benefits of the standing position

concerns regarding airway stability, portability of equipment (e.g. the use of portable ventilators), management of multiple attachments and a reduced level of monitoring once the bed space has been left. Some degree of monitoring is vital in terms of titrating the appropriate intensity level, along with monitoring of the patients physiological response, to ensure the safety of these interventions. Portable pulse oximeters and the Borg breathlessness scale provide quick and simple methods of achieving this. This progression in mobility is an essential part of supporting long-term recovery, with higher mobility levels within ICU associated with reduced hospital length of stay and improved functional status at the point of hospital discharge [26, 27].

6.3.3 Considerations

Alongside physical improvements, a number of other factors need to be considered to help guide the progression of mobility. Given the complex nature of early rehabilitation in patients with multi-organ failure, close multidisciplinary team working and collaboration are essential to success. This can be supported through the implementation of rehabilitation ward rounds. These rounds provide team members with the opportunity to discuss the patients' rehabilitation in the context of medical stability, any current plan for weaning of sedation and respiratory support, management of delirium and to highlight other team member tasks which may require completion [36]. This process allows for a comprehensive consideration of the balance between the patient's physiological reserve and any weaning from mechanical ventilation. In addition, the patient's ability to mobilise at any given time can be affected by a number of factors such as fluctuations in underlying condition, nutritional status, sleep quality or motivation levels. An understanding regarding the intensity of exercise is, therefore, a key requirement to ensure rehabilitation plans are individualised and dynamic in response to changing patient requirements.

6.3.4 Challenging Situations

The process of sitting on the edge of the bed can at times be labour intensive, particularly for patients who are obese, of low arousal or with profound ICU-AW, where it may take four or even five members of staff to transfer the patient to the edge of the bed. Alternatively, factors such as a poorly tolerated airway, multiple attachments including positional femoral lines, low dose inotropic support or postural hypotension may raise safety concerns around the process of moving a patient onto the edge of the bed. In these instances, stretcher chairs can be used, providing a safe and controlled method of assessing or mobilising these patients. Devices such as these can allow earlier transfer out of bed for patients deemed to be high risk [37], allowing safe and supportive seating positions to be achieved gradually. This is particularly useful in those patients with postural hypotension or reduced consciousness levels. Passive chair transfer is also useful for those patients with low physiological reserve, being significantly less demanding than sitting on the edge of the bed [38]. In these early stages, sitting should be limited to a maximum of 1 h to prevent the risk of developing pressure ulcers or becoming overly fatigued.

For patients with a reduced conscious level, postural hypotension or those not ready to commence more active rehabilitation, tilt tables can be used to facilitate early standing. This provides an excellent method of increasing arousal whilst facilitating weight-bearing through the lower limbs, preventing joint contractures and improving lower limb strength. Straps to support the knees and trunk make this a very stable position, with the addition of head support recommended for those patients with a low conscious levels to maintain a more supported posture. In the case of low arousal or postural hypotension, the device should be tilted gradually in 10-degree increments whilst keeping a close eye on the patient's blood pressure.

This can be monitored using the inclinometer in the underside of the device. Once the point at which hypotension begins to develop is noted (systolic BP <90 mmHg or MAP <60 mmHg), it is recommended to lower the degree of tilt by 5–10° and select this as the starting treatment position of choice. This level should then be documented in the patients' treatment record and set as a target to achieve or surpass at the next session. Where possible, active exercise, particularly of the lower limbs, can also be added to treatment sessions to support circulation and venous return.

The supported standing position can also be utilised for more alert patients who still have limited sitting balance and are unable to stand independently. The full tilt position allows an upright standing position to be achieved much earlier with a number of benefits. As well as those listed above, the addition of functional or reaching tasks squats can also be considered to start to challenge dynamic balance and reciprocal trunk activity. As patients progress, there is also the option to remove the knee support to allow knee bends/squats using the patient's own weight as a source of resistance training. This can be commenced at lower inclines and such as 30° in the early stages, increasing the degree of tilt and hence the effect of gravity as the patients progress.

6.4 How to Measure Patient and Service Outcomes

The evaluation of a patient's physical function in the ICU is needed for a variety of reasons and can be examined at different stages of critical illness. Measuring physical function early and longitudinally in the ICU will identify those at risk of poor outcomes and, therefore, which patients may require more targeted rehabilitation interventions [39]. Additionally, it will provide ongoing information on patients' recovery trajectory and the efficacy of the rehabilitation interventions employed, guiding modification of intervention. Understanding a patients' pre-admission status through proxy or patient reporting (e.g. Clinical Frailty Scale or WHO Disability Assessment Schedule 2.0) will also direct appropriate rehabilitation goals [40].

There are several different outcome measures available for use in ICU that measure a variety of different aspects of physical function across the three constructs of the World Health Organisation (WHO) ICF framework [41]. The three constructs of the ICF framework are body function and structure (anatomical and physiological structure), activities (specific task completion in a controlled environment) and participation (completion of a task in the context of an everyday environment/situation). The ICF framework recognises that function is affected through a combination of an individual's health condition and personal and environmental factors. Therefore, the evaluation of distinct aspects of physical function in ICU will not necessarily correlate with limitations in activities and participation [42].

There are several factors to consider when choosing an outcome measure. The purpose of the assessment of physical function will dictate which outcome measure is most appropriate. If the aim is to evaluate a rehabilitation intervention, then the measure should reflect the domain of the ICF framework that the intervention is targeting. Therefore, if an intervention is aimed at increasing patient mobility, then an outcome measure focused on mobility should be used (e.g. ICU Mobility Scale or Manchester Mobility Score). As most physical function outcome measures are dependent on the patient's effort, the feasibility of each outcome measure should also be considered based on individual patients' physical and mental capacity. Finally, the time, training and resources of each outcome measure should be considered in the context of the local ICU rehabilitation service. Some outcome measures require additional equipment (e.g. Chelsea Critical Care Physical Assessment Tool) or more time to assess multiple domains (e.g. Functional Status Score for the ICU) that may make them more difficult to complete locally.

Measures of physical function can also be used to evaluate rehabilitation provision at a service level. Tracking the physical outcome measure results for the ICU population (or subgroup) over a period may indicate the efficacy of the rehabilitation service; however, this needs to be reviewed in the context of the many other factors present on ICU that affect the patients' physical function. Recording rehabilitation-specific patient milestones may be a more accurate way of evaluating the effectiveness of a rehabilitation service. These can include time from admission to first rehabilitation assessment, active rehabilitation intervention or mobilisation out of bed. This could even be as simple as recording the patient level of mobility on discharge from ICU. This simple measure can provide vital information to both evaluate current mobility level but also stratify those patients most at risk, and therefore in need of rehabilitation. Recovery trajectory is significantly impacted by the patients physical function or mobility level at the point of ICU discharge [43, 44]. Patients unable to stand at the point of ICU discharge are most likely to miss rehabilitation sessions, spend longer times in hospital and are more likely to require ongoing rehabilitation in the community after hospital discharge [14, 45, 46].

Although mobilisation in ICU is feasible, there are many institutional, clinician and patient barriers to implementation [47]. The use of standardised outcome measures and good governance practices can identify and overcome some of these barriers. Accurately recording any adverse events that may occur either during or as a result of rehabilitation interventions will allow any safety concerns to be quickly identified and potentially address apprehensions within the wider ICU team. Further evaluation of the service against clinical guidelines [29] will also identify areas of compliance and non-compliance with current best practice.

To further develop an ICU rehabilitation service, it is fundamental that the rehabilitation currently being delivered is accurately recorded. This may include the number and duration of interventions, number and profession of staff required and the content of the intervention. It is also important to evaluate who the rehabilitation interventions are being delivered to, i.e. the complexity of the patient. This can be evaluated by severity of illness, mode of ventilation and method of delivery, presence of advanced cardiovascular support or renal replacement therapy.

Understanding what is currently being delivered will allow for identification of the unmet rehabilitation need within the ICU and can be tracked to changes in service performance over time. This provides the context in terms of changes in patient caseload or complexity, and staffing. Unmet rehabilitation need could take the form of delays or missed rehabilitation assessments or interventions.

6.5   ICU Discharge to the Ward

Even in units with established programmes of early mobilisation, around 50% of patients are discharged from ICU unable to stand or transfer to a chair [27]. Despite these low levels seen at ICU discharge, patient mobility levels actually continue to decrease in the days following step down to the ward [48]. This problem is further exacerbated due to a lack of cohorting of these patients, who instead are spread throughout the wards in a hospital depending on the original speciality of their underlying admission. This results in a wide spread, both geographically and in the underlying skills of the receiving wards, meaning post-ICU care commonly misses key patient needs. This is often compounded by limited provision of rehabilitation in the ward environment with patients receiving physiotherapy an average two times per week [45]. This is a result of factors such as competing priorities, where competition for care occurs on the ward due to a focus on patient flow and the need to prirotise care for those patients identified for hospital discharge. To ensure seamless transition between areas, it is therefore vital that handover documentation between ICU and wards should be in written form, standardised and structured [49, 50]. This should include information regarding the patients current goals and indicualised rehabilitation plan.

6.6   Discharge from the Hospital, What Happens Next?

Survivors of critical illness frequently experience long-term physical impairment, persistent exercise limitation and decreased health-related quality of life (QoL) [12]. The subsequent socioeconomic burden of critical illness is also high. Patients report significant healthcare utilisation after discharge from hospital, with up to half of patients re-admitted to the hospital at least once in the first year after discharge [51]. Rates of return to employment following admission to ICU are also extremely low, with up to a third of patients not returning to work within 5 years of ICU admission [52].

Despite the high level of physical impairment following critical illness, the provision of rehabilitation following discharge from the hospital is inconsistent and with no clear evidence to guide details of what should be delivered or which patients it should be delivered to [53]. Expert recommendations suggest that goals of rehabilitation programmes following discharge from hospital should aim to increase functional exercise capacity, aerobic capacity, skeletal and respiratory muscle strength, activities of daily living (ADL) function, QoL, and understanding of Post-Intensive Care Syndrome (PICS) and recovery [54]. The programmes should also aim to decrease pain. The recommendations for interventions to be included in the rehabilitation programme are wide ranging and include interval or endurance cardiovascular training, high-intensity interval training, functional exercises, strengthening exercises, inspiratory and expiratory respiratory muscle training and patient and family education [54].

Many of the post-hospital rehabilitation interventions employed are based on the successful supervised group exercise programmes used in cardiac and pulmonary rehabilitation, constituting cardiopulmonary and general strengthening exercises along with education. These have been delivered over 6–7 weeks in an outpatient setting with patients undertaking additional unsupervised exercise at home. Group-based exercise interventions have demonstrated improvements in anxiety, depression and physical function, and exercise capacity when combined with nutritional supplementation [55, 56]. However, attendance at group-based exercise programmes can be variable and depend greatly on both the location of the hospital and the size of the area it serves. Similar rehabilitation interventions have been delivered on an individual basis, both at home and in an outpatient setting, with improvements in patient balance and anxiety [57, 58].

When developing a post-hospital rehabilitation programme, it is important to also consider what patients feel to be beneficial or not. Patients and their relatives have reported that they feel their rate of recovery is accelerated by rehabilitation following hospital discharge and that supervised exercise was a key facilitator of this perceived benefit [59]. However, they have also identified pre-existing physical limitations and mental health as barriers to exercise, with patients finding it difficult to continue to exercise following the completion of their rehabilitation programme because of a lack of self-motivation.

The delivery of a post-hospital discharge rehabilitation programme for survivors of critical illness should be tailored to the individual hospital and patient requirements. To maximise the success of a rehabilitation programme, it is important to first address any pre-existing conditions that the patient may have, which will involve liaising with other clinical specialties. The heterogeneous nature of the ICU population means that patients will benefit most from individualised rehabilitation. This can take to form of group based or 1:1 intervention but should involve supervised exercise (as this has been identified as a key component by patients) and be delivered over a minimum of 6 weeks. To ensure that patients participate in the rehabilitation programme and then continue with unsupervised exercise, it is important to discover what individual patients' motivators are and develop goals based on these. Finally, each contact with ICU patients after discharge from hospital is important; therefore, patients should be provided with education on their recovery at every opportunity.

6.7   Conclusion

From the moment, a patient is admitted to critical care they are deteriorating from a physical perspective. The longer the associated period of immobility, the poorer the long-term physical, functional and psychological outcomes. Collaborative multidisciplinary team working is essential to support programmes of early mobilisation, particularly for those patients most at risk. These programmes are guided by expert consensus and national guidelines to ensure both the safety of commencing mobilisation and its progression. Whilst starting rehabilitation early is key to improving both short- and long-term patient outcomes, this forms only part of the journey and it is essential that services are structured to support ongoing rehabilitation following hospital discharge.

Key Take Home Messages

- Survivors of critical illness experience significant physical and non-physical morbidity.
- Early mobilisation is safe and feasible for patients, even in the acute phases of critical illness.
- Early and structured mobilisation has the potential to improve both patient and organisational outcomes.
- Close MDT working, structure and consistency are key to success.
- Patients often have significant ongoing rehabilitation needs following hospital discharge.

References

1. Puthacheary Z, Rawal J, Mcphail M, et al. Acute skeletal muscle wasting in critical illness. JAMA. 2013;310:1591–600.
2. Dirks ML, Wall BT, van de Valk B, Holloway TM, Holloway GP, Chabowski A, et al. One week of bed rest leads to substantial muscle atrophy and induces whole-body insulin resistance in the absence of skeletal muscle lipid accumulation. Diabetes. 2016;65(10):2862–75.
3. Batt J, Dos Santos CC, Cameron JI, Herridge MS. Intensive care unit-acquired weakness: clinical phenotypes and molecular mechanisms. Am J Respir Crit Care Med. 2013;187:238–46.
4. Stevens RD, Marshall SA, Cornblath DR, et al. A framework for diagnosing and classifying intensive care unit-acquired weakness. Crit Care Med. 2009;37:S299–308.
5. Chohan S, Ash S, Senior L. A team approach to the introduction of safe early mobilisation in an adult critical care unit. BMJ. 2018;7(4):e000339.
6. Hespel P, Op't Eijnde B, Van Leemputte M, et al. Oral creatine supplementation facilitates the rehabilitation of disuse atrophy and alters the expression of muscle myogenic factors in humans. J Physiol. 2001;536:625–33.
7. Veldhuizen JW, Verstappen FT, Vroeme JP, et al. Functional and morphological adaptations following four weeks of knee immobilization. Int J Sports Med. 1993;14:283–7.
8. De Jonghe B, Bastuji-Garin S, Durand MC, et al. Respiratory weakness is associated with limb weakness and delayed weaning in critical illness. Crit Care Med. 2007;35:2007–15.
9. Garnacho-Montero J, Amaya-Villar R, Garcia-Garmendia JL, et al. Effect of critical illness polyneuropathy on the withdrawal from mechanical ventilation and the length of stay in septic patients. Crit Care Med. 2005;33:349–54.
10. Griffiths RD, Hall JB. Intensive care unit-acquired weakness. Crit Care Med. 2010;38:779–87.
11. Griffiths J, Hatch RA, Bishop J, et al. An exploration of social and economic outcome and associated health related quality of life after critical illness in general intensive care unit survivors: a 12-month follow-up study. Crit Care. 2013;17(3):R100.
12. Herridge MS, Tansey CM, Matte A, et al. Functional disability 5 years after acute respiratory distress syndrome. N Engl J Med. 2011;364(14):1293–304.
13. Medrinal C, Prieur G, Bonnevie T, Gravier FE, Mayard D, Desmalles E, Smondack P, Lamia B, Combret Y, Fossat G. Muscle weakness, functional capacities and recovery for COVID-19 ICU survivors. BMC Anesthesiol. 2021;21(1):64. https://doi.org/10.1186/s12871-021-01274-0.

14. McWilliams D, Weblin J, Hodson J, Veenith T, Whitehouse T, Snelson C. Rehabilitation levels in patients with COVID-19 admitted to intensive care requiring invasive ventilation. An observational study. Ann Am Thorac Soc. 2021;18(1):122–9. https://doi.org/10.1513/AnnalsATS.202005-560OC.

15. Levine S, Nguyen T, Taylor N, et al. Rapid disuse atrophy of diaphragm fibres in mechanically ventilated humans. N Engl J Med. 2008;358:1327–35.

16. Vorona S, Sabatini U, Al-Maqbali S, Bertoni M, Dres M, Bissett B, et al. Inspiratory muscle rehabilitation in critically ill adults: a systematic review and meta-analysis. Ann Am Thorac Soc. 2018;15(6):735–44.

17. Jung B, Moury PH, Mahul M, et al. Diaphragmatic dysfunction in patients with ICU-acquired weakness and its impact on extubation failure. Intensive Care Med. 2016;42:853–61.

18. Truong AD, Fan E, Brower RG, Needham DM. Bench to bedside review: mobilizing patients in the intensive care unit—from pathophysiology to clinical trials. Crit Care. 2009;13:1–8.

19. Convertino VA, Bloomfield SA, Greenleaf JE. An overview of the issues: physiological effects of bed rest and restricted physical activity. Med Sci Sports Exerc. 1997;29:187–90.

20. Kashihara H, Haruna Y, Suzuki Y, et al. Effects of mild supine exercise during 20 days bed rest on maximal oxygen uptake rate in young humans. Acta Physiol Scand. 1994;616:19–26.

21. Owen HC, Vanhees I, Solie L, Roberts SJ, Wauters A, Luyten FP, Van Cromphaut S, Van den Berghe G. Critical illness-related bone loss is associated with osteoclastic and angiogenic abnormalities. J Bone Miner Res. 2012;27(7):1541–52.

22. Zerwekh JE. The effects of twelve weeks of bed rest on bone histology, biochemical markers of bone turnover, and calcium homeostasis in eleven normal subjects. J Bone Miner Res. 1998;13(10):1594–601.

23. Rawal J, et al. A pilot study of change in fracture risk in patients with acute respiratory distress syndrome. Crit Care. 2015;19(1):165.

24. Parker A, Sricharoenchai T, Needham DM. Early rehabilitation in the intensive care unit: preventing physical and mental health impairments. Curr Phys Med Rehabil Rep. 2013;1(4):307–14.

25. Morris PE, Berry MJ, Files DC, Thompson JC, Hauser J, Flores L, et al. Standardized rehabilitation and hospital length of stay among patients with acute respiratory failure. JAMA. 2016;315(24):2694–9.

26. Schweickert W, Pohlman MC, Pohlman AS, Nigos C, Pawlik AJ, Esbrook CL, et al. Early physical and occupational therapy in mechanically ventilated, critically ill patients: a randomised controlled trial. Lancet. 2009;373:1874–82.

27. McWilliams D, Weblin J, Atkins G, et al. Enhancing rehabilitation of mechanically ventilated patients in the intensive care unit: a quality improvement project. J Crit Care. 2015;30(1):13–8.

28. Nydahl P, Sricharoenchai T, Chandra S, Sari KF, Huang M, Fischill M, et al. Safety of patient mobilization and rehabilitation in the intensive care unit. Systematic review with meta-analysis. Ann ATS. 2017;14(5):766–77. https://doi.org/10.1513/AnnalsATS.201611-843SR.

29. National Institute for Health and Care Excellence (NICE). Rehabilitation after critical illness. London: NICE. (Nice guideline no. 83); 2009.

30. Devlin JW, Yoanna S, Gelinas C, et al. Clinical practice guidelines for the prevention and management of pain, agitation/sedation, delirium, immobility, and sleep disruption in adult patients in the ICU. Crit Care Med. 2018;46(9):1532–48.

31. Adler J, Malone D. Early mobilization in the intensive care unit: a systematic review. Cardiopulm Phys Ther. 2012;23(21):5–13.

32. Arias-Fernandez P, Romero-Martin M, Gomez-Salgado J, Fernandez-Garcia D. Rehabilitation and early mobilisation in the critical care patient: systematic review. J Phys Ther Sci. 2018;30:1193–201.

33. Hodgson CL, Stiller K, Needham DM, et al. Expert consensus and recommendations on safety criteria for active mobilization of mechanically ventilated critically ill adults. Crit Care. 2014;18(6):658.

34. Parry S, Puthucheary Z. The impact of extended bed rest on the musculoskeletal system in the critical care environment. Extreme Physiol Med. 2015;4:16.

35. Winkleman C. Bed rest in health and critical illness—a body systems approach. AACN Adv Crit Care. 2009;20(3):254–66.
36. Bakhru R, McWilliams DJ, Wiebe DJ, Spuhler VJ, Schweickert WD. Intensive care unit structure variation and implications for early mobilization practices: an international survey. Ann Am Thorac Soc. 2016;13(9):1527–37.
37. McWilliams D, Atkins G, Hodson J, Snelson C. The Sara Combilizer as an early mobilisation aid for critically ill patients: a prospective before and after study. Aust Crit Care. 2017;30(4):189–95.
38. Collings N, Cusack R. A repeated measures, randomized cross-over trial, comparing the acute exercise response between passive and active sitting in critically ill patients. BMC Anesthesiol. 2015;15:1.
39. Parry SM, Huang M, Needham DM. Evaluating physical functioning in critical care: considerations for clinical practice and research. Crit Care. 2017;21(1):249.
40. Jolley SE, Bunnell AE, Hough CL. ICU-acquired weakness. Chest. 2016;150(5):1129–40.
41. Stucki G. International classification of functioning, disability, and health (ICF): a promising framework and classification for rehabilitation medicine. Am J Phys Med Rehabil. 2005;84(10):733–40.
42. Needham DM, Wozniak AW, Hough CL, Morris PE, Dinglas VD, Jackson JC, et al. Risk factors for physical impairment after acute lung injury in a national, multicenter study. Am J Respir Crit Care Med. 2014;189(10):1214–24.
43. Herridge MS, et al. The RECOVER program: disability risk groups and 1-year outcome after 7 or more days of mechanical ventilation. Am J Respir Crit Care Med. 2016;194(7):831–44.
44. Iwashyna TJ. Trajectories of recovery and dysfunction after acute illness, with implications for clinical trial design. Am J Respir Crit Care Med. 2012;186(4):302–4.
45. Gustafson OD, et al. A human factors analysis of missed mobilisation after discharge from intensive care: a competition for care? Physiotherapy. 2021;113:6.
46. Mcwilliams D, et al. Is the Manchester mobility score a valid and reliable measure of physical function within the intensive care unit. ICM Exp. 2015;3(Suppl 1):7.
47. Parry SM, Nydahl P, Needham DM. Implementing early physical rehabilitation and mobilisation in the ICU: institutional, clinician, and patient considerations. Intensive Care Med. 2018;44(4):470–3.
48. Hopkins RO, et al. Physical therapy on the wards after early physical activity and mobility in the intensive care unit. Phys Ther. 2012;92(12):1518–23.
49. Stelfox HT, et al. A multi-center prospective cohort study of patient transfers from the intensive care unit to the hospital ward. Intensive Care Med. 2017;43:1485–94.
50. Boyd JM, et al. Administrator perspectives on ICU-to-ward transfers and content contained in existing transfer tools: a cross-sectional survey. J Gen Intern Med. 2018;33:1738–45.
51. Batchelor A. Getting it right first time—adult critical care; 2021.
52. Kamdar BB, Sepulveda KA, Chong A, Lord RK, Dinglas VD, Mendez-Tellez PA, et al. Return to work and lost earnings after acute respiratory distress syndrome: a 5-year prospective, longitudinal study of long-term survivors. Thorax. 2018;73(2):125–33.
53. Connolly B, Salisbury L, O'Neill B, Geneen L, Douiri A, Grocott MP, et al. Exercise rehabilitation following intensive care unit discharge for recovery from critical illness. Cochrane Database Syst Rev. 2015;(6):CD008632.
54. Major ME, Kwakman R, Kho ME, Connolly B, McWilliams D, Denehy L, et al. Surviving critical illness: what is next? An expert consensus statement on physical rehabilitation after hospital discharge. Crit Care. 2016;20(1):354.
55. McWilliams DJ, Benington S, Atkinson D. Outpatient-based physical rehabilitation for survivors of prolonged critical illness: a randomized controlled trial. Physiother Theory Pract. 2016;32(3):179–90.
56. Jones C, Eddleston J, McCairn A, Dowling S, McWilliams D, Coughlan E, Griffiths RD. Improving rehabilitation after critical illness through outpatient physiotherapy classes and essential amino acid supplement: a randomized controlled trial. J Crit Care. 2015;30(5):901–7.

57. McDowell K, O'Neill B, Blackwood B, Clarke C, Gardner E, Johnston P, et al. Effectiveness of an exercise programme on physical function in patients discharged from hospital following critical illness: a randomised controlled trial (the REVIVE trial). Thorax. 2017;72(7):594–5.
58. Battle C, James K, Temblett P, Hutchings H. Supervised exercise rehabilitation in survivors of critical illness: a randomised controlled trial. J Intensive Care Soc. 2019;20(1):18–26.
59. Ferguson K, Bradley JM, McAuley DF, Blackwood B, O'Neill B. Patients' perceptions of an exercise program delivered following discharge from hospital after critical illness (the revive trial). J Intensive Care Med. 2017;34:978.

Infection Prevention and Control: Simple Measures, Challenging Implementation

7

Sonia O. Labeau, Stijn I. Blot, Silvia Calviño-Günther, Elena Conoscenti, and Mireia Llauradó Serra

7.1   Introduction

Intensive care unit (ICU) professionals use their full range of expertise into ensuring the best of care for the critically ill patients admitted to their unit and safeguarding them from adverse events that might compromise their short- and long-term outcomes. A common adverse event in the ICU is the development of healthcare-associated infection (HAI). As the impact of HAI on patient outcomes can be detrimental, infection prevention is of key importance for patients to be discharged in a timely and successful way.

S. O. Labeau (✉)
Department of Internal Medicine and Pediatrics, Ghent University, Ghent, Belgium

School of Healthcare, Nursing programme, HOGENT University of Applied Sciences and Arts, Ghent, Belgium
e-mail: sonia.labeau@hogent.be

S. I. Blot
Department of Internal Medicine and Pediatrics, Ghent University, Ghent, Belgium
e-mail: stijn.blot@ugent.be

S. Calviño-Günther
CHU Grenoble Alpes, Réanimation Médicale Pôle Urgences Médecine Aiguë,
Grenoble, France

E. Conoscenti
Direction of Healthcare Professions, ISMETT IRCCS UPMC, Palermo, Italy
e-mail: econoscenti@ismett.edu

M. L. Serra
Faculty of Medicine and Health Sciences, Nursing Department, Universitat Internacional de
Catalunya, Barcelona, Spain
e-mail: mllaurados@uic.es

Infection prevention and control is, however, far too broad a topic to be discussed in a comprehensive way in a short chapter. Those interested can find extensive guidance on setting up and conducting evidence-based, effective and efficient programs in the World Health Organisation's (WHO) recently updated *Guidelines on core components of infection prevention and control programme* [1]. Their soundly written publication can be considered as recommended, if not required reading for each healthcare professional committed to the battle against HAI. This chapter will confine itself to concisely presenting the problem of HAI, as well as the basic infection prevention principles and current evidence-based guidelines for the prevention of the *Big Four* infections in the adult ICU. Health professionals' limited compliance with infection prevention guidelines is discussed, as well as the evidence for interventions to optimize guideline adherence.

7.2 Healthcare-Associated Infection in the ICU

Healthcare-associated infections are frequent complications in the ICU. This section concisely delineates their epidemiology and impact, and stresses the value of evidence-based infection prevention for timely and successfully discharging patients from the ICU.

7.2.1 Definitions and Impact

HAI is defined as infection occurring in a patient during the process of care in a healthcare facility and considered ICU-acquired if it occurs in the ICU after more than 48 h from admission [1]. According to overall European estimates, HAI annually leads to 16 million extra days of hospital stay, 37,000 attributable deaths, and important unfavourable psychosocial patient outcomes [1, 2]. As the annual economic impact in Europe is as high as €7 billion [1], the financial consequences to both patients and the healthcare system are overwhelming.

7.2.2 The Big Four

The so-called *Big Four* infection types accounting for over 80% of all HAIs in the ICU are ventilator-associated pneumonia (VAP), central line-associated bloodstream infection (CLABSI), catheter-associated urinary tract infection (CAUTI), and surgical site infection (SSI) [3]. European data collected in 2019 among patients staying in the ICU for more than 2 days revealed a mean device-adjusted rate of 7.8 episodes per 1000 intubation days for VAP, of 3.4 episodes per 1000 central venous catheter (CVC) days for CLABSI and of 2.8 episodes per 1000 urinary catheter days for CAUTI [4].

7.2.2.1 VAP

VAP is defined as pneumonia developing more than 48–72 h after intubation and is the most frequent nosocomial infection in the ICU [5]. Although the attributable mortality remains a matter of debate, its rate was reported to be between 10% and 13% in recent reviews and meta-analysis [6, 7].

VAP results from the microbial invasion of the normally sterile lung parenchyma. Oropharyngeal or tracheobronchial colonization with pathogenic bacteria starts with microorganisms adhering to epithelial cells in the patient's upper and lower airway; the stomach has also been proposed as an important reservoir. In the absence of adequate infection control procedures, bacteria can additionally gain entry into the lower respiratory tract through inhalation of aerosols generated primarily by contaminated nebulization devices. Gram-negative aerobes comprise the majority of infections [5].

The presence of an artificial airway is estimated to cause a 21-fold increase in the patient's risk of developing pneumonia. Additional risk factors (Table 7.1) increase the chance of the respiratory tract being colonized with pathogens and predispose to the aspiration of contaminated fluids and secretions [5–7].

7.2.2.2 CLABSI

The main complication resulting from the use of intravascular catheters is blood-stream infection. When there is a formal confirmation of the association between the catheter and the bloodstream infection, the term *catheter-related bloodstream infection* is used. In case the association is lacking but the patient's central catheter is the most likely source of the bloodstream infection, the condition is defined as CLABSI [8]. A 2015 meta-analysis investigating the attributable mortality from 18 studies—of which 17 involved ICU patients—found a 2.75 odds ratio (95% confidence interval [CI], 1.86–4.07) of in-hospital death associated with CLABSI [9].

As illustrated by Fig. 7.1, CLABSI can originate from four mechanisms.

Table 7.1 Risk factors for VAP development

Impaired host defences/increased aspiration	Large inoculum of organisms	Overgrowth of virulent organisms
Endotracheal tubes	Bacterial colonization	Prolonged antibiotic use
Nasogastric tubes	Gastric alkalinization	Prior antibiotic exposure
Enteral feeding tubes	Iatrogenic	Iatrogenic
Reintubation	Sinusitis	Central venous catheters
Tracheostomy	Malnutrition	Comorbid illness
Supine positioning	Contaminated respiratory equipment	Frequent hospitalizations
Impaired mental status		Prolonged hospital stay
Sedation		
Transport of mechanically ventilated patient out of ICU		
Surgery		

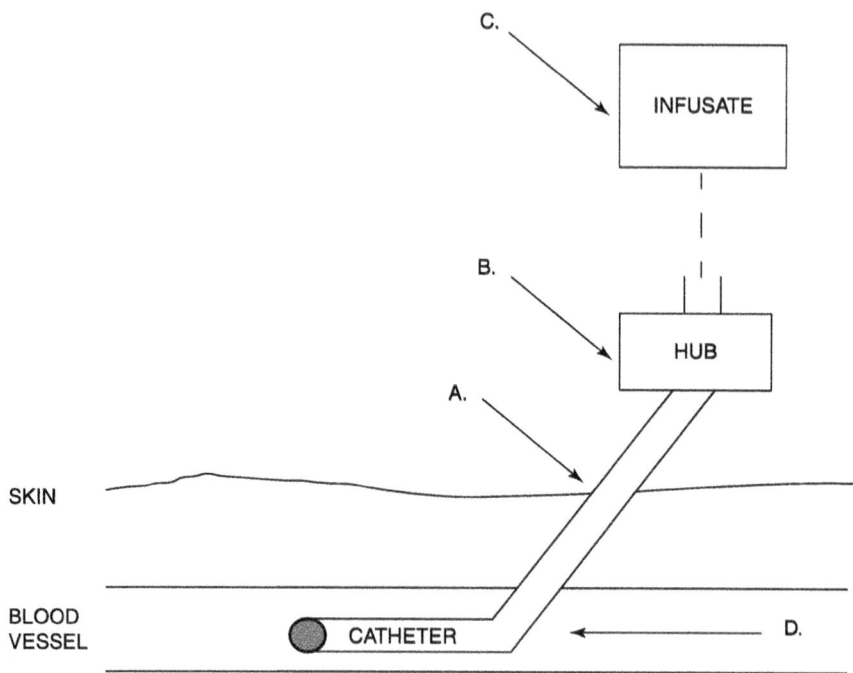

Fig. 7.1 Pathogenesis of CLABSI

Of these four mechanisms, bacteria colonizing the skin site (A) are the most frequent cause of catheter infection, followed by colonization and subsequent infection of catheter hubs (B). The organisms involved in these processes may be endogenous and belong to the patient's normal skin flora, or exogenous and originate from clinicians' hands or contaminated disinfectants. Contamination of infusate (C) and haematogenous seeding from bacteraemia (D) are rather infrequent causes. Bacteria attached to the catheter can produce a biofilm, which is a slime layer composed of glycoproteins such as fibrinogen, fibronectin, collagen and laminin, and that allows bacteria, particularly Staphylococci, to attach even more easily to the catheter [8].

The risk of CLABSI in ICU patients is high and varies with the reason for catheter use, type of intravascular catheter, as well as with the catheter's dwell time, with the highest incidence densities for non-tunnelled short-term CVCs [10].

7.2.2.3 CAUTI

CAUTI refers to microorganisms having invaded the bladder of a patient with an indwelling catheter, and is most often asymptomatic. The presence of a urethral catheter bypasses natural defence mechanisms which normally prevent interactions between bacteria and the epithelial cells of the urinary tract and inhibits the mechanical wash-out effect of the urinary stream. Biofilm production between the catheter and the urethral mucosa additionally provides a favourable environment for bacterial invasion and proliferation. As a result, micro-organisms entering the urinary tract are able to multiply to dangerous levels in as short a time as one single day [11].

At the time of catheter insertion, micro-organisms inhabiting the meatus or distal urethra can contaminate the catheter tip and subsequently be introduced directly into the bladder, or contamination can occur from breaches in asepsis during the insertion procedure. During catheterization, extraluminal contamination occurs by microorganisms ascending from the perineum or the urethral meatus. Intraluminal contamination in turn results from the reflux of bacteria from a contaminated drainage bag or catheter-drainage tube junction. Even with meticulous attention to the maintenance of the closed system, the space between the external catheter and the urethral mucosa offers opportunities for bacterial entry directly into the bladder [12].

As 12–16% of adult patients have a urinary catheter at some time during hospitalization and as the daily risk of acquiring bacteriuria with an indwelling catheter is 3–7%, the cumulative burden of CAUTI is substantial [12] .

7.2.2.4 SSI

Surgical site infections (SSIs) rank as one of the most prevalent healthcare-associated infections (HAIs), leading to extended post-operative hospitalisation, supplementary surgical interventions, and elevated mortality rates [13]. SSIs are classified into (a) superficial incisional, involving the skin and the subcutaneous tissue; (b) deep incisional, involving deep soft tissues such as the fascial and muscle layers of the incision and (c) organ/space SSI, involving any part of the anatomy other than the incised body wall layers that was opened or manipulated during surgery [14, 15].

Causative pathogens usually originate from the patient's endogenous flora and locally contaminate the surgical site during surgery. Alternatively, they may originate from remote preoperative infections, particularly in prosthesis or other implant surgery, or from exogenous sources such as surgical team members, the operating theatre environment and materials used during the procedure [15, 16]. The risk of SSI can be outlined as (*dose of bacterial contamination* ∗ *virulence*)/*resistance of the host.*

Last publications by the ECDC for 2018–2020 in Europe reported 19,680 SSI from a total of 255,958 surgical procedures for 9 different types of surgical procedures followed-up. Incidence density percentages had large variations depending on type of surgical procedure, from 0.6% for knee prothesis operations to 9.5% in open colon surgery. Consistently, laparoscopic procedures in both cholecystectomy and colon operations had lower percentages of SSIs and incidence density than open procedures [13]. Nevertheless, when comparing 2020 to the years 2018–2019, a reduction in the annual count of surgical procedures was observed, as well as a decrease in the number of countries reporting data to the ECDC.

7.3   The ICU Is the Hospital's Hot Zone for HAI

The reasons why the majority of HAI are acquired in the ICU are numerous. First, critically ill patients are particularly susceptible to infection due to underlying conditions and comorbidities, and to impaired immunity induced by their condition or medications. Next, they are exposed to multiple invasive devices that bypass their protective barriers and may be inserted in emergency situations with compromised aseptic technique. Finally, multidrug-resistant organisms increasingly make the ICU the most dangerous hospital environment for their dissemination and potential patient to patient transmission [1].

An analysis of 2 European point prevalence studies including 310,755 patients in 28 countries found at least 1 HAI in 19.2% of ICU patients compared with 5.2% on average for all other specialties combined [17]. The problem is most pronounced in low and middle-income countries with a pooled overall HAI density in adult ICUs of 47.9 per 1000 patient-days [18].

7.4   Prevention Works!

Timely diagnosis and appropriate management have been shown to improve patient outcomes; however the focus remains on preventing infections from developing. A recent meta-analysis assessing the proportion of HAIs prevented by multifaceted infection control interventions found an overall 35–55% potential for decreasing HAI rates. The risk of bias was, however, high in 143 of the 144 studies included [3].

HAI rates have significantly decreased throughout Europe between 2008 and 2012. The incidence of VAP was reduced from 13.6 to 10.2 episodes per 1000 intubation days (p <0.001); of CLABSI from 3.6 to 3.0 episodes per 1000 CVC days (p = 0.001) and of CAUTI from 4.9 to 4.1 per 1000 urinary catheter days (p <0.001) [19]. Additionally, today's literature abounds with successes booked in HAI prevention in the ICU. These inspiring and encouraging reports clearly illustrate that sustained and evidence-based prevention efforts are rewarding and fully worth investing in.

7.4.1   Basics of Infection Prevention

Worldwide, there is a constant search for novel approaches to prevent HAIs, often involving the newest technologies. It should, however, not be forgotten that all efforts must always build on a number of long established key foundations to have a chance of being successful.

7.4.1.1 Standard and Transmission-Based Precautions
The CDC Standard Precautions, updated in 2022, include recommendations on correct and timely hand hygiene practices, appropriate personal protective equipment, respiratory hygiene and cough etiquette, sharps safety and safe injection practices, cleaning, disinfection, and sterilization of medical equipment and on adequate environmental infection prevention and control [20].

As a result of multiple adaptations by several agencies and organisations, legitimate concern has however been raised that healthcare professionals might no longer have a common understanding of the term *Standard Precautions* and what exactly is included [21]. In this context, it is important to always keep in mind that the most recent version of the CDC guideline remains the preeminent reference.

7.4.1.2 Hand Hygiene: Cornerstone of Infection Prevention and Control

Of all basics of infection prevention, hand hygiene is the single most important practice to reduce the transmission of infectious agents in healthcare settings [22]. Transmission of pathogens from one patient to another most frequently occurs through contaminated hands of healthcare professionals. Infected or draining wounds, sputa and other body secretions are well-known reservoirs, but pathogens are also commonly recovered from intact patient skin and the inanimate patient and hospital environment. Defective hand cleansing results in inadequate hand decontamination, which in turn may lead to both within- and between-patient cross-contaminations [23].

7.4.1.3 Principles for Preventing All Device-Related Infections

In a worldwide sample of patients admitted to ICUs in September 2017 (1150 centers in 88 countries), the prevalence of suspected or proven infection was as high as 54%, and 70% of these patients were receiving at least 1 antibiotic. Patients with proven or suspected infection had a substantial risk of in-hospital mortality, at about 30% [22]. Due to critically ill patients' debilitated condition, several invasive devices are required for monitoring and/or treatment purposes, even though they are well known to be significant risk factors for infection [24]. As such, it is not surprising that three HAIs out of the *Big Four*, namely VAP, CLABSI and CAUTI, are associated with the use of invasive devices.

Figure 7.2 illustrates the basic principles for the prevention of all device-related infections and Table 7.2 summarizes the translation of these principles into practice for VAP, CLABSI and CAUTI.

Fig. 7.2 Principles for preventing device-associated infections

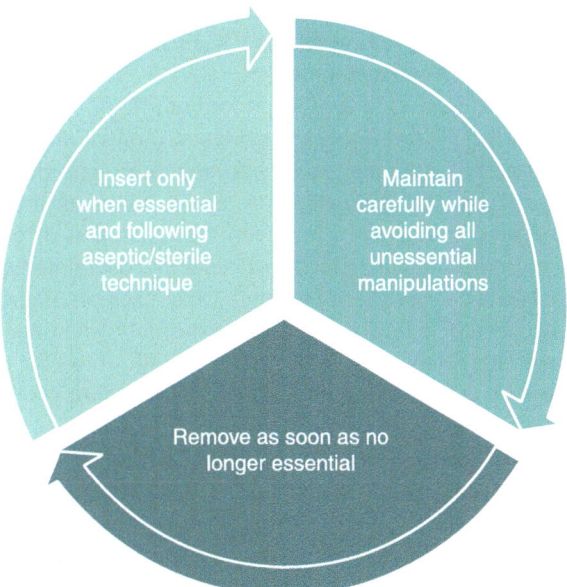

Table 7.2 Principles applied to VAP, CLABSI and CAUTI

VAP [7, 25]	CLABSI [8]	CAUTI [11]
Avoid intubation/replace by noninvasive ventilation if possible	Use aseptic techniques and maximal sterile barriers during catheter insertion	Insert upon strict indication only and consider alternatives to indwelling catheters
Change ventilator circuits only if visibly soiled or malfunctioning	Promptly replace catheters inserted during an emergency	Secure indwelling catheters properly
Comply with CDC guidelines for sterilization and disinfection of respiratory care equipment	Select CVCs appropriately as to intended purpose and duration of use and with the essential number of ports or lumens only	Use aseptic techniques and the smallest bore catheter possible upon catheter insertion
Daily, combine spontaneous breathing and awakening trials	Evaluate and manage insertion sites daily and appropriately	Maintain a closed drainage system and do not replace catheters and bags routinely
	Assess the need for the catheter daily and remove as soon as no longer essential	Assess the need for the catheter daily and remove as soon as no longer essential

7.4.2 Evidence-Based Guidelines for Preventing the Big Four

Besides the aforementioned general principles, specific guidelines are available for the prevention of each of the *Big Four*.

7.4.2.1 Which Guideline to Follow?

Since the rise of the concept of evidence-based medicine in the early 1990s, health-care agencies worldwide have been investing considerable efforts in guideline development and dissemination.

In the field of infection prevention, the CDC and WHO are the main global authorities. However, also numerous professional societies, local organizations, healthcare institutions and even individual care units have issued guidelines and best practice recommendations. The result of all these well-intended and labour-intensive initiatives is, however, a proliferation of guidelines of varying quality, some even containing inconsistencies and contradicting recommendations.

Healthcare professionals may experience problems when being faced with the challenge of guideline selection, especially when not fully familiar with the concepts of evidence-based care. Table 7.3 illustrates the multitude of available guidelines by providing a non-comprehensive overview of recommendations issued for the prevention of CLABSI in the last 6 years only.

In the absence of guidance by their hospital's Infection Control Committee or institutional experts, individual healthcare professionals are advised to determine their choice on the basis of two considerations: (1) who is the publisher of the guideline and (2) which is the most recent guideline. Guidelines issued by authoritative international health agencies such as the CDC and WHO may safely be considered

Table 7.3 CLABSI prevention guidelines issued since 2014

Agencies	
US Centres for Disease Control and Prevention	Recommendations on the use of chlorhexidine-impregnated dressings for prevention of intravascular catheter-related infections: an update to the 2011 guidelines for the prevention of intravascular catheter-related infections from the Centres for Disease Control and Prevention, 2017 Guidelines for the Prevention of Intravascular Catheter-Related Infections, 2011, updated July 2017
Professional societies	
• Society for Healthcare Epidemiology of America/ Infectious Diseases Society of America	• Septimus EJ. Society for Healthcare Epidemiology of America Compendium updates 2022. Curr Opin Infect Dis. 2023 Jun 1. https://doi.org/10.1097/QCO.0000000000000926. Epub ahead of print. PMID: 37260268
Asia Pacific Society of Infection Control	Executive Summary: APSIC guide for the prevention of Central Line Associated Bloodstream Infections, 2016 Full guidance: APSIC guide for the prevention of central line associated bloodstream infections, 2015
Association for Professionals in Infection Control and Epidemiology	Guide to Preventing Central Line-Associated Bloodstream Infections. Implementation Guide, 2015
Canadian Patient Safety Institute	Central Line-Associated Bloodstream Infection: Getting Started Kit, 2019
National/Regional Institutes (Europe only)	
Denmark: Statens Serum Institut	National infection control guidelines for use of intravascular catheters, 2016
Germany: Robert Koch InstiTute, Commission for Hospital Hygiene and Infection Prevention	Prevention of vascular catheter-associated infections, 2017
Ireland: Royal College of Physicians	Prevention of Intravascular Catheter-related Infection in Ireland. Update of 2009 National Guidelines, 2014
Netherlands: Dutch National Institute for Public Health and the Environment	Phlebitis and bloodstream infections due to intravenous infusion catheters, 2015
United Kingdom: UK Department of Health United Kingdom: Health Protection Scotland	Epic3: National Evidence-Based Guidelines for Preventing Healthcare-Associated Infections in NHS Hospitals in England, 2014 Compendium of HAI guidance; page 34, 2019 Preventing infections when inserting and maintaining a central vascular catheter, 2014
France: French Society of Intensive Care Medicine (SRLF), French-Speaking Group of Paediatric Emergency Rooms and Intensive Care Units (GFRUP) and the French-Speaking Association of Paediatric Surgical Intensivists (ADARPEF)	Timsit JF, Baleine J, Bernard L, et al. Expert consensus-based clinical practice guidelines management of intravascular catheters in the intensive care unit. *Ann Intensive Care.* 2020;10(1):118. Published 2020 Sep 7. https://doi.org/10.1186/s13613-020-00713-4

(continued)

Table 7.3 (continued)

Spain: Spanish Society of Infectious Diseases and Clinical Microbiology and (SEIMC) and the Spanish Society of Spanish Society of Intensive and Critical Care Medicine and Coronary Units (SEMICYUC)	Chaves F, Garnacho-Montero J, Del Pozo JL, et al. Diagnosis and treatment of catheter-related bloodstream infection: Clinical guidelines of the Spanish Society of Infectious Diseases and Clinical Microbiology and (SEIMC) and the Spanish Society of Spanish Society of Intensive and Critical Care Medicine and Coronary Units (SEMICYUC). *Med Intensiva (Engl Ed)*. 2018;42(1):5–36. https://doi.org/10.1016/j.medin.2017.09.012
Italy: AMCLI Associazione Microbiologi Clinici Italiani ETS (AMCLI ETS)	Diagnostic Pathway for circulatory system infections 2023. Percorso Diagnostico INFEZIONI DEL TORRENTE CIRCOLATORIO 2023

credible and of excellent quality, while the most recently published guidelines have the biggest chance of including the most recent insights. References to the most recent guidelines for the prevention of VAP [11, 12], CLABSI [8, 26–29], CAUTI [11, 12], and SSI [14–16, 30, 31] are in the reference list.

7.4.2.2 Healthcare Professionals' Adherence to the Recommendations Is Low

Evidence-based prevention strategies may only be effective over prolonged periods when integrated into the behaviour of all staff involved in patient care. Unfortunately, adherence to infection prevention and control recommendations is known to be low, even though many of the procedures are of low-complexity.

As such, the simple task of sustainably adhering to hand hygiene recommendations seems to be a persistent, universal challenge, even though hand hygiene is considered an essential practice, foundational to any health-care associated infection program, and recommendations are regularly updated [32]. Compliance rates in the ICU are as low as 30–40%, which is even lower than the already disappointing rates registered in general hospital settings (50–60%) [33]. These figures, obtained by direct observation and thereby already potentially biased, are moreover in stark contrast to the over 70% self-estimated rates of performance reported by healthcare professionals [34], thus suggesting a massive misjudgement of the problem.

Rello et al. investigated physicians' adherence to evidence-based guidelines for VAP prevention and found an overall self-reported non-adherence rate of 37% [35]. Ricart et al. used the same questionnaire in a sample of ICU nurses and found the non-adherence rate to be 22.3% [36]. Similar findings, usually obtained by self-reporting, are abundantly reported for all evidence-based guidelines for preventing the *Big Four*. As self-reports on behaviour are often coloured by social desirability bias, it can be presumed that the actual non-adherence rates are even higher.

7.4.2.3 Barriers to Adherence

Numerous research has been focusing on identifying the risk factors, beliefs and attitudes associated with non- or low compliance with recommendations.

In the context of hand hygiene, the majority of self-reported reasons for non-adherence are related to organisational factors including lack of time, of appropriate agents for hand hygiene, and lack of sinks and alcoholic hand rub dispensers or their inconvenient location. In addition presumed skin damage caused by alcohol-based hand rub remains an important barrier [35].

In the context of adherence to VAP guidelines, disagreement with the interpretation of clinical trials (35%), unavailability of resources (31.3%) and costs (16.9%) were the most common self-reported reasons for non-adherence in the aforementioned study by Rello et al. [35], while the ICU nurses surveyed by Ricart and colleagues [36] considered patient-related barriers to be significantly more important (1.8% vs. 8.2%, odds ratio 4.87; 95% CI 2.90–8.18). Healthcare professionals may also become discouraged by the excess of sometimes unattractively presented, hard-to-read information, and lose their confidence in guidelines in general when being confronted with inconsistencies [37]. Moreover lack of knowledge of the guidelines has been recognized as an elemental barrier to adherence [38–41]. Generally, when addressing infection control barriers to adherence, it has been previously emphasized that every organisation should identify the underlying causes within the context of the local culture and environment [42]. Figure 7.3 offers an overview of the most commonly reported reasons for non-adherence.

7.4.2.4 Strategies to Improve Guideline Adherence

Various strategies to enhance healthcare professionals' adherence have been tested, with varying degrees of success. An illustrative example is the Agency for Healthcare Research and Quality (AHRQ), which has introduced a toolkit for ICUs aimed at enhancing infection control. This toolkit provides a comprehensive approach to reduce CLABSI and CAUTI rates, offering assessments, implementation strategies, and solutions for addressing common challenges [43].

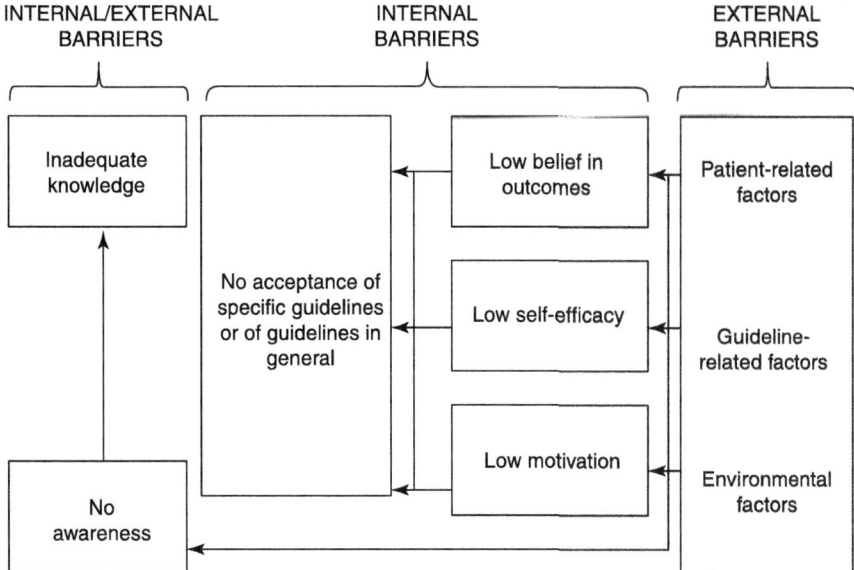

Fig. 7.3 Barriers to guideline adherence: schematic overview

A systematic review of 38 studies published since 2009 on interventions to improve hand hygiene compliance in the ICU, including coercion, education, enablement, environmental restructuring, providing incentives, modelling, persuasion, restriction and finally, training, merely concluded that best evidence-based practice for improving compliance in ICU settings remains unestablished today [44]. Another recent review conducted by Clancy et al. analysing clinical trials from 2014 to 2020 reached a similar conclusion, as both single interventions and multi-modal strategies revealed only modest to moderate improvements in hand hygiene compliance [45]. Even though the last 20 years have seen an impressive interest on hand hygiene literature, with a spectacular peak during the COVID-19 pandemic outbreak, when alcohol-based hand rub was proved effective against the SARS-CoV-2 virus, compliance has yet to be improved. The WHO remains actively engaged promoting hand hygiene best practices organising in 2021 the Technical Advisory Group in order to evaluate the scientific aspects of hand hygiene and define a research agenda for the next 5 years [46]. Interestingly, recent research illustrated objective knowledge alone might not be sufficient; it has to be integrated and subjectively believed in, in order to transform compliance and practice [47, 48].

Strategies and bundled interventions have proven effective in both raising adherence to evidence-based prevention of the *Big Four* and reducing infection rates were the subjects of a systematic review of 71 studies published between 2006 and 2012. Across all four infections, a moderate strength of evidence suggested that both adherence and infection rates improve when either audit and feedback combined with provider reminder systems or audit and feedback alone are added to the basic strategies of organizational change and provider education [49].

Provider education was identified by a plethora of studies as of key value for the promotion of guideline adherence and is currently considered an essential prerequisite for successful guideline implementation [16, 50–55]. As such, staff education has been integrated as a basic and fixed component in all HAI prevention guidelines [7, 12, 26–28], including different types of teaching approaches, from the basic paper-based self-study or in-person workshop approach, to modular, spaced teaching in combination with a series of games or case studies [56].

While awaiting further guidance from research:

1. each and every healthcare worker's professional and moral standards should be intrinsic drivers to take personal responsibility for sustained adherence to infection prevention and control recommendations;
2. managers should be attentive for signs of hand hygiene fatigue among staff;
3. implementation strategies should be chosen that have at least a certain grade of evidence promoting their use, are tailored to the unit, supported by the entire ICU team;

4. monitoring and evaluating compliance with hand hygiene and overall infection prevention recommendations should be considered a priority in each ICU to create and foster a culture of safety;
5. as evidenced by a systematic review on interventions aimed at reducing catheter-associated urinary tract infections, directing efforts toward motivational, social, and environmental influences could enhance the design and effectiveness of any interventions [57].

7.5   Conclusions

The ICU is the hospital's hot zone for infection, with VAP, CLABSI, CAUTI and SSI as the four most prevailing healthcare-associated infections in this setting. The long established basics of infection prevention remain of paramount importance today. High adherence to recommendations is pivotal to prevention of HAI and to facilitate a timely and smooth ICU discharge instead of facing an unnecessary increased ICU stay with all the inherent associated risks.

An overwhelming body of evidence supports the key importance of appropriate and evidence-based infection prevention and control, and the success of sustained prevention efforts to significantly reduce infection rates.

Prevention efforts may only be effective over sustained periods if they are integrated into the behaviour of all staff members involved in patient care. Selection of strategies promoting guideline adherence and implementation should be based on whether they have at least a certain grade of evidence promoting their use, are tailored to the unit, and are supported by the entire ICU team. Simultaneously, monitoring and evaluating compliance with hand hygiene and overall infection prevention recommendations should be considered an ever-lasting priority in each ICU.

Lastly, each and every healthcare worker's high professional and moral standards should be important drivers for taking personal responsibility to sustainably adhere to infection prevention and control recommendations to promote safe and timely discharge for the ICU patient.

Key Take Home Messages
- HAI is a common adverse event in the ICU, associated with important unfavourable patient and economic outcomes.
- The *Big Four* infections in the adult ICU are VAP, CLABSI, CAUTI and SSI.
- An estimated 35–55% of HAIs is preventable if multifaceted, evidence based prevention strategies are applied.
- Sustained adherence to basic infection prevention strategies combined with specific evidence based recommendations is key to successfully prevent HAI and thus to facilitate a timely and smooth ICU discharge.

References

1. World Health Organization. Guidelines on core components of infection prevention and control programmes at the national and acute health care facility level. Geneva: World Health Organization; 2016. https://iris.who.int/handle/10665/251730. Accessed 3 Nov 2023.
2. Currie K, Melone L, Stewart S, et al. Understanding the patient experience of health care-associated infection: a qualitative systematic review. Am J Infect Control. 2018;46(8):936–42. https://doi.org/10.1016/j.ajic.2017.11.023.
3. Schreiber PW, Sax H, Wolfensberger A, Clack L, Kuster SP, Swissnoso. The preventable proportion of healthcare-associated infections 2005–2016: systematic review and meta-analysis. Infect Control Hosp Epidemiol. 2018;39(11):1277–95. https://doi.org/10.1017/ice.2018.183.
4. European Centre for Disease Prevention and Control. Annual epidemiological reports (AERs). Published online October 27, 2023. https://www.ecdc.europa.eu/en/publications-data/monitoring/all-annual-epidemiological-reports.
5. Chastre J, Fagon JY. Ventilator-associated pneumonia. Am J Respir Crit Care Med. 2002;165(7):867–903. https://doi.org/10.1164/ajrccm.165.7.2105078.
6. Papazian L, Klompas M, Luyt CE. Ventilator-associated pneumonia in adults: a narrative review. Intensive Care Med. 2020;46(5):888–906. https://doi.org/10.1007/s00134-020-05980-0.
7. Klompas M, Branson R, Eichenwald EC, et al. Strategies to prevent ventilator-associated pneumonia in acute care hospitals: 2014 update. Infect Control Hosp Epidemiol. 2014;35(S2):S133–54. https://doi.org/10.1017/S0899823X00193894.
8. O'Grady NP, Alexander M, Burns LA, et al. Guidelines for the prevention of intravascular catheter-related infections. Am J Infect Control. 2011;39(4):S1–34. https://doi.org/10.1016/j.ajic.2011.01.003.
9. Ziegler MJ, Pellegrini DC, Safdar N. Attributable mortality of central line associated bloodstream infection: systematic review and meta-analysis. Infection. 2015;43(1):29–36. https://doi.org/10.1007/s15010-014-0689-y.
10. Zingg W, Walder B, Pittet D. Prevention of catheter-related infection: toward zero risk? Curr Opin Infect Dis. 2011;24(4):377–84. https://doi.org/10.1097/QCO.0b013e32834811ed.
11. Gould CV, Umscheid CA, Agarwal RK, Kuntz G, Pegues DA, Healthcare Infection Control Practices Advisory Committee (HICPAC). Guideline for prevention of catheter-associated urinary tract infections 2009. Infect Control Hosp Epidemiol. 2010;31(4):319–26. https://doi.org/10.1086/651091.
12. Lo E, Nicolle LE, Coffin SE, et al. Strategies to prevent catheter-associated urinary tract infections in acute care hospitals: 2014 update. Infect Control Hosp Epidemiol. 2014;35(Suppl 2):S32–47.
13. ECDC. Annual epidemiological report for 2018–2020 healthcare-associated infections: surgical site infections. Published online May 2023. https://www.ecdc.europa.eu/sites/default/files/documents/Healthcare-associated%20infections%20-%20surgical%20site%20infections%20 2018-2020.pdf.
14. Berríos-Torres SI, Umscheid CA, Bratzler DW, et al. Centers for Disease Control and Prevention guideline for the prevention of surgical site infection, 2017. JAMA Surg. 2017;152(8):784–91. https://doi.org/10.1001/jamasurg.2017.0904.
15. Mangram AJ, Horan TC, Pearson ML, Silver LC, Jarvis WR. Guideline for prevention of surgical site infection, 1999. Centers for Disease Control and Prevention (CDC) Hospital Infection Control Practices Advisory Committee. Am J Infect Control. 1999;27(2):97–132; quiz 133–134; discussion 96.
16. World Health Organization Global guidelines for the prevention of surgical site infection. 2nd ed. Geneva: World Health Organization; 2018. Accessed 3 Nov 2023. https://iris.who.int/handle/10665/277399.
17. Suetens C, Latour K, Kärki T, et al. Prevalence of healthcare-associated infections, estimated incidence and composite antimicrobial resistance index in acute care hospitals and long-

term care facilities: results from two European point prevalence surveys, 2016 to 2017. Euro Surveill. 2018;23(46):1800516. https://doi.org/10.2807/1560-7917.ES.2018.23.46.1800516.
18. Allegranzi B, Nejad SB, Combescure C, et al. Burden of endemic health-care-associated infection in developing countries: systematic review and meta-analysis. Lancet. 2011;377(9761):228–41. https://doi.org/10.1016/S0140-6736(10)61458-4.
19. ECDC. European Centre for Disease Prevention and Control Incidence and attributable mortality of healthcare-associated infections in intensive care units in Europe. Published online 2018. 2018. https://www.ecdc.europa.eu/en/publications-data/incidence-and-attributable-mortality-healthcare-associated-infections-intensive.
20. Siegel JD, Rhinehart E, Jackson M, Chiarello L, Health Care Infection Control Practices Advisory Committee. 2007 guideline for isolation precautions: preventing transmission of infectious agents in health care settings. Am J Infect Control. 2007;35(10 Suppl 2):S65–164. https://doi.org/10.1016/j.ajic.2007.10.007.
21. Curran ET. Standard precautions: what is meant and what is not. J Hosp Infect. 2015;90(1):10–1. https://doi.org/10.1016/j.jhin.2014.12.020.
22. Vincent JL, Sakr Y, Singer M, et al. Prevalence and outcomes of infection among patients in intensive care units in 2017. JAMA. 2020;323(15):1478–87. https://doi.org/10.1001/jama.2020.2717.
23. World Health Organization. WHO patient safety. WHO guidelines on hand hygiene in health care. Geneva: World Health Organization; 2009. (WHO/IER/PSP/2009/01):262.
24. Vincent JL, Rello J, Marshall J, et al. International study of the prevalence and outcomes of infection in intensive care units. JAMA. 2009;302(21):2323–9. https://doi.org/10.1001/jama.2009.1754.
25. Torres A, Niederman MS, Chastre J, et al. International ERS/ESICM/ESCMID/ALAT guidelines for the management of hospital-acquired pneumonia and ventilator-associated pneumonia: guidelines for the management of hospital-acquired pneumonia (HAP)/ventilator-associated pneumonia (VAP) of the European Respiratory Society (ERS), European Society of Intensive Care Medicine (ESICM), European Society of Clinical Microbiology and Infectious Diseases (ESCMID) and Asociación Latinoamericana del Tórax (ALAT). Eur Respir J. 2017;50(3):1700582. https://doi.org/10.1183/13993003.00582-2017.
26. Marschall J, Mermel LA, Fakih M, et al. Strategies to prevent central line-associated bloodstream infections in acute care hospitals: 2014 update. Infect Control Hosp Epidemiol. 2014;35(Suppl 2):S89–107.
27. Perin DC, Erdmann AL, Higashi GDC, Sasso GTMD. Evidence-based measures to prevent central line-associated bloodstream infections: a systematic review. Rev Lat Am Enfermagem. 2016;24:e2787. https://doi.org/10.1590/1518-8345.1233.2787.
28. Velasquez Reyes DC, Bloomer M, Morphet J. Prevention of central venous line associated bloodstream infections in adult intensive care units: a systematic review. Intensive Crit Care Nurs. 2017;43:12–22. https://doi.org/10.1016/j.iccn.2017.05.006.
29. CDC. 2017 updated recommendations on the use of chlorhexidine-impregnated dressings for prevention of intravascular catheter-related infections. Published online July 17, 2017. https://www.cdc.gov/infectioncontrol/pdf/guidelines/c-i-dressings-H.pdf.
30. Ban KA, Minei JP, Laronga C, et al. American College of Surgeons and Surgical Infection Society: surgical site infection guidelines, 2016 update. J Am Coll Surg. 2017;224(1):59–74. https://doi.org/10.1016/j.jamcollsurg.2016.10.029.
31. NICE. Surgical site infections: prevention and treatment. Published online August 19, 2020. https://www.nice.org.uk/guidance/NG125.
32. Glowicz JB, Landon E, Sickbert-Bennett EE, et al. SHEA/IDSA/APIC practice recommendation: strategies to prevent healthcare-associated infections through hand hygiene: 2022 update. Infect Control Hosp Epidemiol. 2023;44(3):355–76. https://doi.org/10.1017/ice.2022.304.
33. Erasmus V, Daha TJ, Brug H, et al. Systematic review of studies on compliance with hand hygiene guidelines in hospital care. Infect Control Hosp Epidemiol. 2010;31(3):283–94. https://doi.org/10.1086/650451.

34. Allegranzi B, Sax H, Pittet D. Hand hygiene and healthcare system change within multi-modal promotion: a narrative review. J Hosp Infect. 2013;83(Suppl 1):S3–10. https://doi.org/10.1016/S0195-6701(13)60003-1.

35. Rello J, Lorente C, Bodí M, Diaz E, Ricart M, Kollef MH. Why do physicians not follow evidence-based guidelines for preventing ventilator-associated pneumonia?: a survey based on the opinions of an international panel of intensivists. Chest. 2002;122(2):656–61. https://doi.org/10.1378/chest.122.2.656.

36. Ricart M, Lorente C, Diaz E, Kollef MH, Rello J. Nursing adherence with evidence-based guidelines for preventing ventilator-associated pneumonia. Crit Care Med. 2003;31(11):2693–6. https://doi.org/10.1097/01.CCM.0000094226.05094.AA.

37. Labeau SO, Rello J, Dimopoulos G, et al. The value of E-learning for the prevention of healthcare-associated infections. Infect Control Hosp Epidemiol. 2016;37(9):1052–9. https://doi.org/10.1017/ice.2016.107.

38. Blot SI, Labeau S, Vandijck D, Van Aken P, Claes B, Executive Board of the Flemish Society for Critical Care Nurses. Evidence-based guidelines for the prevention of ventilator-associated pneumonia: results of a knowledge test among intensive care nurses. Intensive Care Med. 2007;33(8):1463–7. https://doi.org/10.1007/s00134-007-0705-0.

39. Labeau SO, Witdouck SS, Vandijck DM, et al. Nurses' knowledge of evidence-based guidelines for the prevention of surgical site infection. Worldviews Evid-Based Nurs. 2010;7(1):16–24. https://doi.org/10.1111/j.1741-6787.2009.00177.x.

40. Labeau SO, Vandijck DM, Rello J, et al. Centers for Disease Control and Prevention guidelines for preventing central venous catheter-related infection: results of a knowledge test among 3405 European intensive care nurses. Crit Care Med. 2009;37(1):320–3. https://doi.org/10.1097/CCM.0b013e3181926489.

41. Labeau S, Vandijck D, Rello J, et al. Evidence-based guidelines for the prevention of ventilator-associated pneumonia: results of a knowledge test among European intensive care nurses. J Hosp Infect. 2008;70(2):180–5. https://doi.org/10.1016/j.jhin.2008.06.027.

42. Anderson R, Rosenberg A, Garg S, et al. Establishing the foundation to support health system quality improvement: using a hand hygiene initiative to define the process. J Patient Saf. 2021;17(1):23–9. https://doi.org/10.1097/PTS.0000000000000578.

43. AHRQ Agency for Healthcare Research and Quality. Toolkit for preventing CLABSI and CAUTI in ICUs. https://www.ahrq.gov/sites/default/files/wysiwyg/hai/tools/clabsi-cauti-icu/clabsi-cauti-icu-report.pdf.

44. Lydon S, Power M, McSharry J, et al. Interventions to improve hand hygiene compliance in the ICU: a systematic review. Crit Care Med. 2017;45(11):e1165–72. https://doi.org/10.1097/CCM.0000000000002691.

45. Clancy C, Delungahawatta T, Dunne CP. Hand-hygiene-related clinical trials reported between 2014 and 2020: a comprehensive systematic review. J Hosp Infect. 2021;111:6–26. https://doi.org/10.1016/j.jhin.2021.03.007.

46. Lotfinejad N, Peters A, Tartari E, Fankhauser-Rodriguez C, Pires D, Pittet D. Hand hygiene in health care: 20 years of ongoing advances and perspectives. Lancet Infect Dis. 2021;21(8):e209–21. https://doi.org/10.1016/S1473-3099(21)00383-2.

47. Wang TJ, Chau B, Lui M, Lam GT, Lin N, Humbert S. Physical medicine and rehabilitation and pulmonary rehabilitation for COVID-19. Am J Phys Med Rehabil. 2020;99(9):769–74. https://doi.org/10.1097/PHM.0000000000001505.

48. Huang A, Hong W, Zhao B, Lin J, Xi R, Wang Y. Knowledge, attitudes and practices concerning catheter-associated urinary tract infection amongst healthcare workers: a mixed methods systematic review. Nurs Open. 2023;10(3):1281–304. https://doi.org/10.1002/nop2.1384.

49. Mauger B, Marbella A, Pines E, Chopra R, Black ER, Aronson N. Implementing quality improvement strategies to reduce healthcare-associated infections: a systematic review. Am J Infect Control. 2014;42(10):S274–83. https://doi.org/10.1016/j.ajic.2014.05.031.

50. Blot S, Koulenti D, Labeau S. Optimizing educational initiatives to prevent ventilator-associated complications. Am J Infect Control. 2017;45(1):102–3. https://doi.org/10.1016/j.ajic.2016.05.035.

51. Labeau SO. Closing the theory-practice gap: a bridge too far? Intensive Crit Care Nurs. 2019;52:61–2. https://doi.org/10.1016/j.iccn.2018.11.006.
52. Labeau SO, Vandijck DM, Vandewoude KH, Blot SI. Obstacles to implementing evidence-based guidelines. Respir Care. 2008;53(4):505–6; author reply 506.
53. Labeau SO. Is there a place for e-learning in infection prevention? Aust Crit Care. 2013;26(4):167–72. https://doi.org/10.1016/j.aucc.2013.10.002.
54. Labeau SO, Vandijck DM, Vandewoude KH, Blot SI. Education reduces ventilator-associated pneumonia rates. Clin Infect Dis. 2008;46(3):479. https://doi.org/10.1086/526344.
55. Tuma P, Vieira Junior JM, Ribas E, et al. A national implementation project to prevent healthcare-associated infections in intensive care units: a collaborative initiative using the breakthrough series model. Open Forum Infect Dis. 2023;10(4):ofad129. https://doi.org/10.1093/ofid/ofad129.
56. Verville L, Dc PC, Grondin D, et al. Using technology-based educational interventions to improve knowledge about clinical practice guidelines. J Chiropr Educ. 2021;35(1):149–57. https://doi.org/10.7899/JCE-19-17.
57. Atkins L, Sallis A, Chadborn T, et al. Reducing catheter-associated urinary tract infections: a systematic review of barriers and facilitators and strategic behavioural analysis of interventions. Implement Sci. 2020;15(1):44. https://doi.org/10.1186/s13012-020-01001-2.

The Power of Communication

8

Jackie McRae, Aeron Ginnelly, Helen Newman, Gemma Clunie, and Mari Viviers

8.1 Speech and Communication Breakdown

Human communication comes in many forms and serves to transmit a message from one person to another or others. Messages may relate to needs, wishes, thoughts and ideas, or perform social functions. Paralinguistic tools such as rate of speech, intonation, volume, body language and facial expression provide nuances and further information to the listener. Context is key to the interpretation of a message [1]. For patients experiencing critical illness, the inability to communicate can be one of the most distressing aspects of admission to ICU [2–4], leading to feelings of fear, anxiety, anger and dehumanisation, and increasing the risk of short- and long-term psychological harm [5–8]. This was particularly highlighted during the

J. McRae (✉)
St George's University of London, London, UK
e-mail: jmcrae@sgul.ac.uk

A. Ginnelly
Critical Care and Neurosciences, Royal Free Hospital, Royal Free London NHS Foundation Trust, London, UK
e-mail: aeron.ginnelly@nhs.net

H. Newman
Critical Care, Respiratory and Surgery, Barnet Hospital, Royal Free London NHS Foundation Trust, London, UK
e-mail: helen.newman3@nhs.net

G. Clunie
Speech and Language Therapy, Therapies Department, Imperial College Healthcare NHS Trust, London, UK
e-mail: gemmaclunie@nhs.net

M. Viviers
St Mary's Hospital, Imperial College NHS Foundation Trust, London, UK
e-mail: mari.viviers@nhs.net

115

COVID-19 pandemic [9–11]. 'Voicelessness' is a term that has been put forward to describe the complex factors involved in ICU-related communication impairment and the effect they bear on patients. Voicelessness encompasses the 'variety of physiological, psychosocial and technological barriers that limit critically ill patients' abilities to represent their thoughts, feelings, desires and needs fully to others' [3].

There are many ways communication can be impaired in patients in ICU. Table 8.1 outlines common causes and mechanisms of communication breakdown.

Table 8.1 Common causes of communication impairment in patients in ICU

Cause	Example	Effect on communication
Artificial airways	Endotracheal tube Tracheostomy	Passes through the oral cavity, pharynx and larynx preventing voicing; reduces intelligibility of mouthing. Increased use of sedation holds means more patients are awake through this [12, 13] Post insertion the cuff is inflated, preventing airflow through the larynx and thus phonation [14] (see below for techniques to restore voice in patients with a tracheostomy)
Acute illness and medication effects	Altered mental state, drowsiness and delirium ICU acquired weakness Drug-induced 'locked-in syndrome' (rare) Dry mouth from mouth breathing, nil-by-mouth status and drug side effects	Affects cognitive-linguistic ability, expressive and receptive language and speech intelligibility Affects up to 80% of ICU patients [15], leads to dysarthria and dysphonia, and can prevent the use of alternative and augmentative communication (AAC, see the following section) Patient is alert and oriented but paralysed and unable to communicate Can be enough to significantly affect speech intelligibility
Underlying diagnoses	Neurological disorders, e.g. stroke, dementia, motor neurone disease and traumatic brain injury Head and neck cancers and treatments Lung conditions, e.g. COPD Vocal fold palsy (due to lung or head and neck cancer, surgery, intubation)	Can lead to impaired speech, language and cognition [16] Can lead to dysphonia and dysarthria [17] May limit sentence length and fluency of speech due to high respiratory rate; frequently associated with dysphonia [18] Causes mild to severe dysphonia [19]
Staffing behaviours	Overly focused on machines and monitors	Supportive behaviours include remaining close, providing reassurance to patients, maintaining eye contact and allowing time for communication to take place. Absence of these is likely to lead to communication breakdown [20]. Training in techniques can increase positive communication interactions and improve staff satisfaction in provision of care [21–24]

Fig. 8.1 Impact of
communication
impairment on patient's
physical, mental and
spiritual well-being

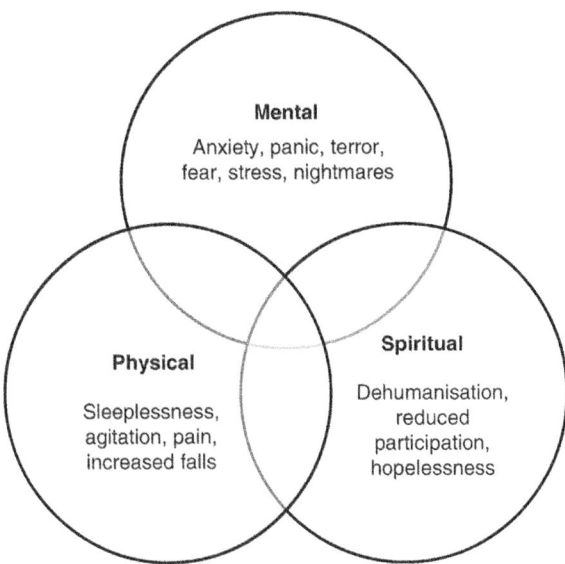

8.1.1   Impact of Communication Impairment on Patients

Voicelessness can have a hugely negative impact on ICU patients [3, 7, 25, 26]. A number of studies report that difficulty speaking is recalled by many patients as the highest ICU-related stressful experience [4] (Fig. 8.1). This lack of voice can have an impact on treatment and decision-making by healthcare staff [3, 26, 27]. Success in communication attempts brings back control, relieves anxiety, restores self-identity and increases staff and patient satisfaction [20, 28–30]. In addition the psychological distress of voicelessness can also contribute to post-ICU syndrome (PICS) [11]. The legacy of the COVID-19 pandemic lives on in the increased awareness and use of personal protective equipment (PPE) such as masks and visors. These PPE measures implemented for staff and patient safety may add an additional layer of challenge to communication interaction for patients with communication impairment in the ICU. In the next section, we will be exploring practical options to support the communication needs of critical care patients.

8.2   Exploring the Impact of Voicelessness

An in-depth understanding of the impact of communication impairment on the patient will aid a humanised and patient-centred approach to critical care [8, 31]. The multidisciplinary team (MDT) should acknowledge that the inability to communicate a person's basic wants, needs and emotions due to 'voicelessness' can be extremely frustrating and creates vulnerability in critical care patients. Meeting the communication needs of voiceless patients is a basic human right, as this experience can lead to mourning the loss of a vital part of what makes the critical care patient human.

8.2.1   Impact of Communication Impairment on the Family and Healthcare Staff

Staff need to be aware of the emotional and physical impact that communication impairment may be having on their patient, including sleeplessness, nightmares and pain, and ensure that daily care routines consider the management of these aspects [32] (Table 8.2). Front-line staff can report feeling unprepared to effectively communicate with patients who have complex communication needs, so this may limit interactions and lead to frustration and stress during daily care routines with patients [33, 34]. ICU nurses have shared their lived experience of caring for patients in ICU with communication impairment due to tracheostomy. These experiences include opposing feelings around communication with these patients as being frustrating, and less motivating but in the same instance feeling satisfaction in supporting these patients [34]. Increased time spent trying to figure out what the patient is trying to communicate may reduce time to deliver interventions or emotional support [35], therefore training for staff can help to build confidence and skills. Istanboulian and Rose [11] recommend that staff should be trained to use multifaceted bundled communication interventions to address the impact of voicelessness, addressing the contextual and individual aspects of the patient and staff as users. Staff should also be able to consider the barriers that may contribute to worsening the impact of voicelessness such as the physical environment, resources, their own skills set and how their own professional identity may shape how they support patients with communication impairment.

A loss of voice and the resulting communication challenges are not only distressing for patients and healthcare staff interacting with them, but for families too. They often experience significant distress when faced with not being able to deduct what their loved one's basic needs and wants are, with more complex messages becoming impossible. Broyles and colleagues [32] reported that families experience a range of emotions and mental health challenges during the time their loved one is in critical care and even directly after discharge from critical care. The loss of their loved one's voice evoked emotions of distress, loss, dismay and frustration [33, 36]. Families experience concern for the patient's safety and vulnerability due to an inability to speak and feel unprepared to deal with communication impairment whilst in the midst of critical illness. In previous studies [32, 36], it has been reported that families are often left on their own to confront the patient's communication challenges and do not always recognise the patient's intact communication capabilities.

Table 8.2 Impact of communication impairment on staff care

Impact on staff care
Unnecessary use of restraint [33]
Misinterpretation of pain or symptoms [35]
Over- or under-treatment [35]
Avoidance of contact [28]
Frustration [28]
Pretend to understand [22]

Therefore, it is crucial that staff effectively engage families to get to know their patient's psychosocial, behavioural and medical history [37] to enable the family members to feel valued and that they are supporting a loved one's social and emotional needs during a period of voicelessness.

8.2.2   Addressing the Impact of Communication Impairment in the ICU

Current practice in critical care is to avoid high sedation levels and to commence rehabilitation earlier for better quality of life and healthcare outcomes [33, 38]. The challenge of communication impairment can be bridged by multidisciplinary involvement and the essential expert services of SLT to guide the family and MDT. To support patients effectively during their journey on the critical care unit, the cascading impact of communication impairment on mental and physical health should be considered in the individualised treatment provided to all intubated patients, or patients with other diagnosis in the ICU that also face communication challenges [8].

The use of multi-level communication interventions should be embedded in a communication strategy and defined in a protocol, supporting the use of low-technology and high-technology alternative and augmentative communication (AAC) options [36]. In cases where family visiting is not possible, measures to mitigate lack of communication and connection with families should be taken, such as virtual visiting. With adequate training and resources, the family and team can support the patient to be involved in care decisions, express levels of pain and strong emotions more easily and raise questions about their medical condition and treatment, improving quality of life and interaction for all involved parties [32, 35]. Family discomfort and lack of proficiency with the use of communication strategies may add to patient's feelings of stress and frustration [32]. When appropriate accommodation for communication challenges is introduced and used by staff and family members, effective symptom management can improve patients' distress and positively impact on health-related quality of life [35]. Practical and effective communication strategies can enable healthcare staff to be proactive rather than reactive in communication engagement with critically ill patients [39] and allow greater participation in their care.

8.2.3   Conclusion

Effective, humanised evidence-based treatment of communication impairment in the ICU has a positive impact on communication efficiency, ventilator weaning, patient affect, accuracy of symptom assessment and treatment, as well as discharge disposition [40]. SLT support in the critical care environment provides an opportunity to guide patients and their families through very stressful circumstances to reach the end goal of more patient autonomy, reduced communication errors and enhanced transfer of accurate information regarding immediate medical and emotional needs [2]. This end goal can be successfully supported by the use of augmentative and alternative communication.

8.3   Alternative and Augmentative Communication Aids

Augmentative and alternative communication (AAC) refers to any communication method, other than oral speech, used to express messages [29]. AAC is vital within a critical care environment to mitigate the impact on patients of not being able to communicate as a result of intubation or tracheostomy. This is particularly true with sedation breaks being used more commonly to improve the outcomes of critically ill patients. The Intensive Care Society recommends that all patients should have access to a range of AAC options to facilitate their rehabilitation [41]. In the wake of the COVID-19 pandemic, access to tablet based technology or simple 'virtual visiting' options has also improved which is a useful adjunct to formal AAC options [10, 42].

AAC methods can be used by patients and caregivers to facilitate the communication of both basic needs and complex information with less frustration than mouthing or gesture [32]. Some AAC can allow the patient to direct conversations, rather than the caregiver needing to provide options (e.g. yes/no questions), thus re-establishing autonomy within the constraints of critical care.

AAC can be broken down into low-technology and high-technology options (Table 8.3). The selection of AAC method depends on a range of factors including:

- Patient status:
  - Level of consciousness
  - Cognition
  - Hearing
  - Vision
  - Language
  - Physical function, e.g. oral motor control, fine motor control
  - Mood
- Staff expertise and time
- Availability of AAC equipment

It should be stressed that the most appropriate choice of AAC for a patient may vary day to day, or hour to hour, based on fluctuations in their status, and that communication support will always be a dynamic and iterative process. A key part of establishing effective AAC also relates to necessary use of PPE since this may limit patient access to certain AAC options, for example lip reading when staff or family are wearing masks. In these cases, alternative options that are acceptable to both patients, staff and family must be explored, alongside simple humanising techniques such as use of body language and visible badges to show who members of the team are.

Table 8.3 Types of AAC (adapted from ten Hoorn and Elbers [29])

No technology	Low technology	High technology
• Mouthing • Gesture • Body language • Eye contact • Response to Y/N questions (head nods, hand squeeze) • Physiological response to stimuli, e.g. intonation, acknowledging presence at bedside (in sedated patients) [43]	• Communication/ picture charts • Eye gaze, e.g. E-tran • Visual analogue scales • Communication books • Alphabet charts • Paper and pen	• Electrolarynx • App-based technology, e.g. mobile phone, tablet, iPad • Eye-gaze technology, e.g. MyTobiiDynavox • LifeVoice communication system (LifeVoice Technologies Inc., USA) • Voice output communication aid (VOCA), e.g. DynaMyte, Lightwriter • PC-based technology, e.g. The Grid2 Package Sensory Software International, UK (eye-gaze and touch screen); ITU talk (used with either switch, trackpad or mouse)

Whenever there is any uncertainty about the best way to support a patient's communication, an expert professional such as a critical care trained SLT should be involved [44]. An algorithm for selecting the most suitable communication aid has been proposed [29] and can support staff in their decisions based on a patient's level of skill to access an aid (Fig. 8.2).

It is valuable to consider the benefits and limitations of a selected AAC device before trialling with a patient, in order to anticipate any challenges that may result in failure and distress (Tables 8.4 and 8.5).

High-tech AAC can be very exciting and appealing to caregivers within a critical care setting, and used well it provides patients with a far more positive and natural communicative option [48, 49]. However, for many of the critical care population, eye gaze or switch technology will not be achievable due to physical or cognitive limitations related either to their underlying diagnosis or the fluctuations in status and mood associated with being critically ill. If high-tech AAC has been identified as worthwhile, for example, for long-term ICU stays this is best set up by expert professionals (ideally by a Specialist AAC MDT, e.g. Compass) as it can then be matched to the individual for maximum success.

8.3.1 Training and Staff Needs in the Critical Care Setting

Low-tech AAC options should be readily available to all caregivers and staff who spend time with the patient with minimal training required to facilitate their use. Pen and paper, communication boards and alphabet charts are easy to produce and store in a critical care setting and can be accessible for all. Similarly, if a patient has a personal high-tech device that they are able to access and use to help them communicate, this should be actively encouraged.

High-tech AAC options will usually require detailed assessment and training by a specialist multidisciplinary team to be used effectively. This can either be completed by expert allied health professionals from the unit particularly if a range of

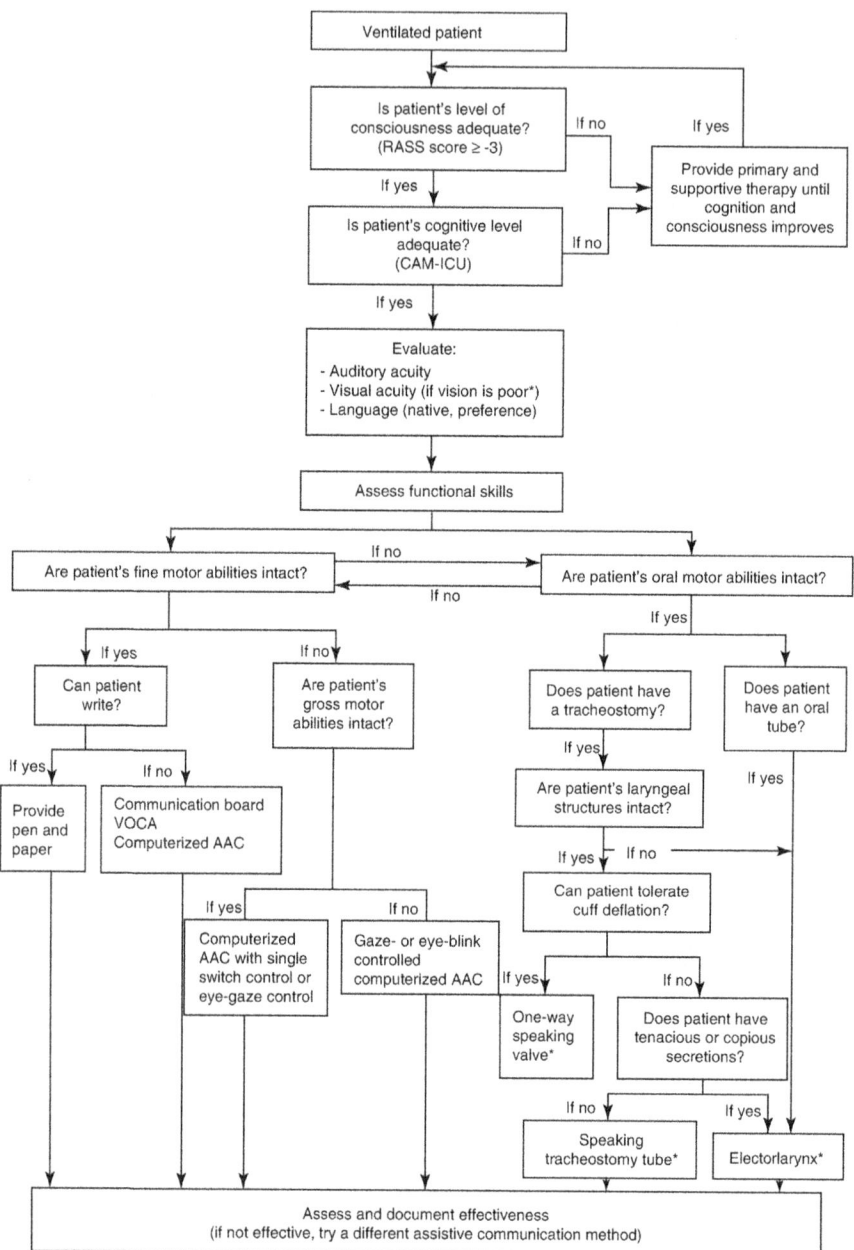

Fig. 8.2 Algorithm for selecting alternative communication methods with intubated patients. *Able to use in patients with poor vision. RASS Richmond Agitation Sedation Scale, CAM-ICU Confusion Assessment Method for the ICU, AAC augmentative and alternative communication, VOCA voice output communication aid. (Reproduced under Attribution 4.0 International (CC BY 4.0) [29])

Table 8.4 Benefits and limitations of low-tech AAC (based on [45, 46])

Type of AAC	Benefits	Limitations
Alphabet charts Communication/ picture charts Visual analogue scales	Easily accessible No need for training or funding Relieve frustration Allow patients to communicate needs Help maintain comfort, dignity and manage pain	Does not allow complex information exchange Requires upper limb and intact visual function to access
Eye gaze, e.g. E-tran board	Relieves frustration Allows patients to communicate needs Helps maintain comfort and dignity and manages pain	Time-consuming Tiring Caregiver and patient need to be confident in its use—element of training required Not suitable for patients with fluctuating conscious level/cognition or difficulties with eye movements
Pen and paper/ whiteboard Communication book	Allow complex information exchange No need for training or funding Relieve frustration Allow patients to communicate needs Help maintain comfort and dignity and manage pain	Not suitable for patients with limited fine motor control or impaired cognition/ language skills

Table 8.5 Benefits and limitations of high-tech AAC

Type of AAC	Benefits	Limitations
Application-based technology, e.g. mobile phone, tablet, iPad®	Inexpensive compared to specialist communication aids Readily available Intuitive and familiar for patients and caregivers [47] Allows complex information exchange through text and images (emojis) Familiar means of communication	Not suitable for patients with limited fine motor control, impaired vision or conscious level Training needed if patient is not familiar with devices/ technology
Eye-gaze technology, e.g. MyTobiiDynavox® (https://www. mytobiidynavox.com)	Suitable for patients with eye movements, consistent level of alertness and cognitive ability but limited gross or fine motor control Allows complex information exchange Potential for stored responses [48] for spontaneous output	Not suitable for patients with limited fine motor control, impaired vision or conscious level Significant training required for caregivers and patient Expensive Tiring

(continued)

Table 8.1 (continued)

Type of AAC	Benefits	Limitations
LifeVoice communication system (LifeVoice Technologies Inc. USA) Voice output communication aid (VOCA), e.g. DynaMyte, Lightwriter PC-based technology, e.g. The Grid2 Package Sensory Software International, UK (eye-gaze and touch screen); ITU talk (used with either switch, trackpad or mouse)	Allows complex information exchange Potential for stored responses [48] and spontaneous communication Switch control can be set up with any body part (fine or gross motor control)	Not suitable for patients with impaired vision or conscious level Significant training required for caregivers and patient Expensive Tiring

high-tech AAC options are available. In certain cases, for example, for patients who are no longer sedated but will require long-term ventilation, have limited physical mobility and are cognitively intact (for example, Guillain–Barré Syndrome), the involvement of a UK Regional Specialised AAC service for individualised AAC set-up is warranted.

In conclusion, specialist SLTs are not only able to support patients, family members and staff in their choice of AAC, but are also key to provide the support and expertise necessary to those patients who are able to make the transition from voiceless to verbal by facilitating speech production. Having a voice during an ICU stay has a significant impact on mental, physical and emotional capacity and recovery leading to a successful ICU discharge and better quality of life [8].

8.4 Facilitating Verbal Communication

For many patients in the ICU setting, the need for prolonged positive pressure ventilation results in them requiring a cuffed tracheostomy tube to be placed. These patients find themselves in a situation where the very tubes that are keeping them alive are restricting their access to a fundamental part of living—the ability to speak.

As seen in the previous section, there are many ways a patient can communicate without needing to access their voice; however for many patients, the most important form of communication is restoration of their own voice, our 'patients want to be heard loud and clear' [50]. In order for humans to produce voice, airflow (from the lungs) is needed to pass through the larynx; this causes the vocal cords to vibrate which in turn produces voice. The voice produced at the level of the vocal cords is then modified by the lips, tongue and soft palate in order to generate speech sounds. When a tracheostomy with an inflated cuff is placed, airflow from the lungs bypasses the larynx (Fig. 8.3), and as such, the patient is not able to produce voice. Despite restoring airflow through the larynx, other factors may have a significant impact on a patient's ability to achieve voice and communicate verbally.

Fig. 8.3 Tracheostomy tube with cuff inflated preventing airflow through larynx to generate voice. (Reproduced with permission from co-author Helen Newman)

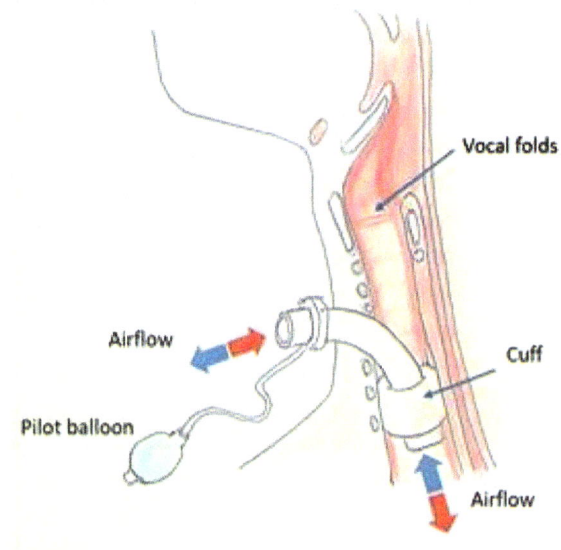

Vocal folds

Airflow

Cuff

Pilot balloon

Airflow

8.4.1   One-Way Valves

One-way valves (traditionally referred to as speaking valves) provide a mechanism to allow expiratory airflow to be diverted around the tracheostomy into the upper airway and through the glottis when the tracheostomy cuff is deflated. Meanwhile, inspiratory airflow can be maintained both through the tracheostomy and the upper airway. There are many different brands of one-way valves available but they all fall into one of two different types: open bias and closed bias valves.

8.4.1.1 Closed Bias Valves

Closed bias valves only open during inspiration and return to a closed position at the end of inspiration; this has the effect of trapping a column of air within the tracheostomy tube thus resulting in no air leak via the diaphragm on the valve [51]. This also results in all of the exhaled air passing up through the upper airway, which facilitates the restoration of Positive End Expiratory Pressure (PEEP) and lung recruitment [52], restoring subglottic pressure [53, 54], restored sensation to laryngeal complex [55] and improving physical mobility [56, 57].

An example of a closed bias one way valve is the Passy-Muir Valve (PMV™). The PMV aqua valve can be used in-line with a ventilator allowing early restoration of voice [58, 59], early assessment of swallow and restoration of oral intake without delaying weaning from the ventilator [60].

8.4.1.2 Open Bias Valves

Unlike closed position valves, open position valves require the patient's exhalatory effort to close the valve. This results in the diaphragm on the valve 'leaking';

therefore, some of the benefits that occur with the closed valve are lost. Patients lose normal levels of subglottic pressure which may reduce cough and ability to manage secretions. These valves cannot be used in line with the ventilator. A number of tracheostomy tube manufacturers produce these valves, for example, Orator Speaking Valve (Portex), Rusch Valve (Rusch) and Shiley™ Speaking Valve (Mallinckrodt).

8.4.1.3 Considerations for One-Way Valve Use

Much research has shown the negative effects of not having a voice can have on patients and given many patients in ICU are limited in their ability to use AAC due to physical weakness and cognitive deficits, the restoration of voice for many of our patients is the most natural and preferred method of communication. As such it is imperative it is prioritised as early as possible [50].

The safe placement of a one-way valve requires specialist assessment by an appropriately skilled MDT in order to optimise voice and respiratory function.

Below are some considerations taken when conducting a one-way valve assessment:

- The cuff must be deflated in order for a one-way valve to be used. If a valve is placed with an inflated cuff the patient will be unable to breath [61].
- Check for upper airway patency, awareness of intubation grade and tracheostomy is tube size is advised. If concerns, consider a brief period of digital occlusion, downsize and/or direct visualisation of upper airway (FNE).
- Check for altered laryngeal responses and impact on secretion management using fibreoptic nasendoscopy.
- Patients should be closely monitored in the early stages with a gradual introduction to valve use.
- When using a one-way valve in-line with a ventilator, adjustments can be made to optimise voice and respiratory comfort whilst wearing a one-way valve. Wallace and McGowan [44] provide a useful trouble-shooting guide on the use of one-way valves for voice restoration in ventilated patients.

Once patients start to generate voice and are able to communicate freely, they often enjoy opportunities to talk to family and friends as well as staff. These sessions should be supervised to ensure safety, adequate ventilation and to reduce fatigue. With regular daily trials, patients using valves have shown improved lung recruitment and ventilator weaning [52].

8.4.2 Leak Speech

By deflating the cuff on the tracheostomy tube, a degree of air will leak through the patient's upper airway and larynx and allowing phonation and voice production (Fig. 8.4). This technique is frequently referred to as 'leak speech'. The quality of voice produced via leak speech may be of poorer quality being breathy and low in volume as expiratory airflow can still exit via the open tracheostomy tube. In some instances, this

Fig. 8.4 Cuff deflation allowing airflow around tracheostomy tube and potential use of a one-way valve for restoration of voice and cough. (Reproduced with permission from co-author, Helen Newman)

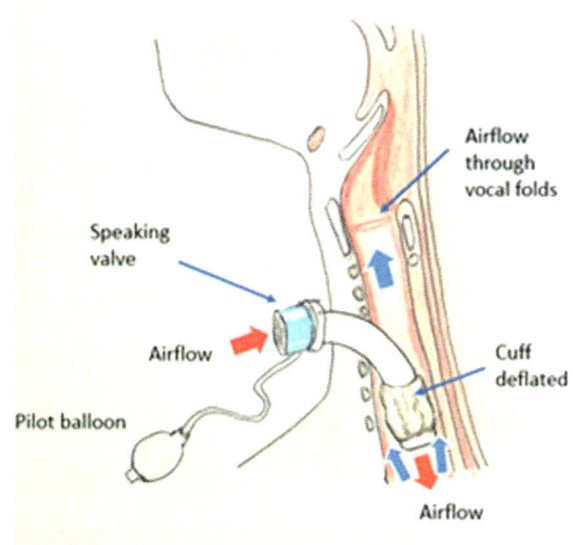

may be acceptable to achieve intelligibility but having an open airway system has implications for losing subglottic pressure that is required for swallowing, and airway protection from secretions, especially to generate a cough [62]. There are a range of options for tube occlusions although evaluation is important to ensure upper airway patency.

8.4.3   Above Cuff Vocalisation (ACV)

In some patients, cuff deflation may not be possible as the level of ventilation required is too high or the risk of aspiration when the cuff is deflated is severe. For this group of patients, a technique known as above cuff vocalisation (ACV) should be considered. Above cuff vocalisation [63] utilises the above cuff suction ports that are now widely available on tracheostomy tubes. The technique works by gas being delivered via the external subglottic port and exiting via the internal port positioned just above the cuff. The airflow then passes through the patient's larynx, allowing phonation without the need for cuff deflation. As the gas being delivered is not humidified, patients can only tolerate this for up to 10–15 min at a time [14]. This technique should only be considered when cuff deflation is not possible due to high ventilation need or unsuccessful trials with valve placement.

8.5   Conclusion

The ability to communicate is of great importance for ICU patients, family and staff. The COVID-19 pandemic created additional challenges to verbal communication with concerns of viral spread, resulting in restricted interventions and lack of family contact. There are a number of verbal and non-verbal options to facilitate communication to enable supported interactions that allow agency and control. An MDT approach is important to ensure focus, consistency and success.

Key Take Home Messages
- Communication is an essential need for patients in ICU and helps humanise care.
- Inflated tracheostomy cuffs stop airflow through the larynx preventing voice.
- Healthcare staff are key to helping restore communication in ICU patients.
- Low-technology and high-technology aids offer alternative means of communication.
- Voice restoration should be considered a priority for our patients.

References

1. van Dijk TA. Discourse and context: a sociocognitive approach. Cambridge: Cambridge University Press; 2008.
2. Radtke JV, Baumann BM, Garrett KL, Happ MB. Listening to the voiceless patient: case reports in assisted communication in the intensive care unit. J Palliat Med. 2011;14(6):791–5.
3. Happ MB. Interpretation of nonvocal behavior and the meaning of voicelessness in critical care. Soc Sci Med. 2000;50(9):1247–55.
4. Pang PSK, Suen LKP. Stressors in the ICU: a comparison of patients' and nurses' perceptions. J Clin Nurs. 2008;17(20):2681–9.
5. Khalaila R, Zbidat W, Anwar K, Bayya A, Linton DM, Sviri S. Communication difficulties and psychoemotional distress in patients receiving mechanical ventilation. Am J Crit Care. 2011;20(6):470–9.
6. Rotondi AJ, Chelluri L, Sirio C, Mendelsohn A, Schulz R, Belle S, et al. Patients' recollections of stressful experiences while receiving prolonged mechanical ventilation in an intensive care unit. Crit Care Med. 2002;30(4):746–52.
7. Bergbom-Engberg I, Haljamae H. Assessment of patients' experience of discomforts during respirator therapy. Crit Care Med. 1989;17(10):1068–72.
8. Newman H, Clunie G, Wallace S, Smith C, Martin D, Pattison N. What matters most to adults with a tracheostomy in ICU and the implications for clinical practice: a qualitative systematic review and metasynthesis. J Crit Care. 2022;72:154145.
9. Scibilia SJ, Gendreau SK, Towbin RT, Happ MB. Impact of COVID-19 on patient-provider communication in critical care: case reports. Crit Care Nurse. 2022;42(4):38–46.
10. Rose L, Yu L, Casey J, Cook A, Metaxa V, Pattison N, et al. Communication and virtual visiting for families of patients in intensive care during the COVID-19 pandemic: a UK National Survey. Ann Am Thorac Soc. 2021;18(10):1685–92.
11. Istanboulian L, Rose L, Yunusova Y, Dale C. Barriers to and facilitators for supporting patient communication in the adult ICU during the COVID-19 pandemic: a qualitative study. J Adv Nurs. 2022;78(8):2548–60.
12. Girard TD, Kress JP, Fuchs BD, Thomason JW, Schweickert WD, Pun BT, et al. Efficacy and safety of a paired sedation and ventilator weaning protocol for mechanically ventilated patients in intensive care (awakening and breathing controlled trial): a randomised controlled trial. Lancet. 2008;371(9607):126–34.
13. Mehta S, Burry L, Cook D, Fergusson D, Steinberg M, Granton J, et al. Daily sedation interruption in mechanically ventilated critically ill patients cared for with a sedation protocol: a randomized controlled trial. JAMA. 2012;308(19):1985–92.
14. UK National Tracheostomy Safety Project. National tracheostomy safety manual. 2013. www.tracheostomy.org.uk.

15. Jolley SE, Bunnell AE, Hough CL. ICU-acquired weakness. Chest. 2016;150(5):1129–40.
16. Brookshire RH, McNeil MR. Introduction to neurogenic communication disorders. 8th ed. St Louis, MO: Mosby; 2015. p. ix, 500-ix, p.
17. Ward EC, van As-Brooks CJ. Head and neck cancer: treatment, rehabilitation, and outcomes. 2nd ed. San Diego, CA: Plural Publishing Inc.; 2014, 640 p.
18. Mohamed EE, El Maghraby RA. Voice changes in patients with chronic obstructive pulmonary disease. Egypt J Chest Dis Tuberc. 2014;63(3):561–7.
19. Rosenthal LH, Benninger MS, Deeb RH. Vocal fold immobility: a longitudinal analysis of etiology over 20 years. Laryngoscope. 2007;117(10):1864–70.
20. Karlsson V, Lindahl B, Bergbom I. Patients' statements and experiences concerning receiving mechanical ventilation: a prospective video-recorded study. Nurs Inq. 2012;19(3):247–58.
21. Happ MB, Sereika SM, Houze MP, Seaman JB, Tate JA, Nilsen ML, et al. Quality of care and resource use among mechanically ventilated patients before and after an intervention to assist nurse-nonvocal patient communication. Heart Lung. 2015;44(5):408–15.e2.
22. Carroll SM. Silent, slow lifeworld: the communication experience of nonvocal ventilated patients. Qual Health Res. 2007;17(9):1165–77.
23. Laerkner E, Egerod I, Olesen F, Hansen HP. A sense of agency: an ethnographic exploration of being awake during mechanical ventilation in the intensive care unit. Int J Nurs Stud. 2017;75:1–9.
24. Alasad J, Ahmad M. Communication with critically ill patients. J Adv Nurs. 2005;50(4):356–62.
25. Freeman-Sanderson AL, Togher L, Elkins M, Kenny B. Quality of life improves for tracheostomy patients with return of voice: a mixed methods evaluation of the patient experience across the care continuum. Intensive Crit Care Nurs. 2018;46:10–6.
26. Morris LL, Bedon AM, McIntosh E, Whitmer A. Restoring speech to tracheostomy patients. Crit Care Nurse. 2015;35(6):13–28.
27. Freeman-Sanderson AL, Togher L, Elkins MR, Phipps PR. Quality of life improves with return of voice in tracheostomy patients in intensive care: an observational study. J Crit Care. 2016;33:186–91.
28. Magnus VS, Turkington L. Communication interaction in ICU—patient and staff experiences and perceptions. Intensive Crit Care Nurs. 2006;22(3):167–80.
29. ten Hoorn S, Elbers PW, Girbes AR, Tuinman PR. Communicating with conscious and mechanically ventilated critically ill patients: a systematic review. Crit Care. 2016;20(1):333.
30. Menzel LK. Factors related to the emotional responses of intubated patients to being unable to speak. Heart Lung. 1998;27(4):245–52.
31. Todres L, Galvin KT, Holloway I. The humanization of healthcare: a value framework for qualitative research. Int J Qual Stud Health Well-being. 2009;4(2):68–77.
32. Broyles LM, Tate JA, Happ MB. Use of augmentative and alternative communication strategies by family members in the intensive care unit. Am J Crit Care. 2012;21(2):e21–32.
33. Happ MB, Garrett KL, Tate JA, Divirgilio D, Houze MP, Demirci JR, et al. Effect of a multi-level intervention on nurse–patient communication in the intensive care unit: results of the SPEACS trial. Heart Lung. 2014;43(2):89–98.
34. Akroute AR, Brinchmann BS, Hovland A, Fredriksen S-TD. ICU nurses' lived experience of caring for adult patients with a tracheostomy in ICU: a phenomenological-hermeneutic study. BMC Nurs. 2022;21(1):214.
35. Tate JA, Sereika S, Divirgilio D, Nilsen M, Demerci J, Campbell G, et al. Symptom communication during critical illness: the impact of age, delirium, and delirium presentation. J Gerontol Nurs. 2013;39(8):28–38.
36. Happ MB, Garrett K, Thomas DD, Tate J, George E, Houze M, et al. Nurse-patient communication interactions in the intensive care unit. Am J Crit Care. 2011;20(2):28–40.
37. Choi J, Tate JA. Evidence-based communication with critically ill older adults. Crit Care Clin. 2021;37(1):233–49.
38. Reschreiter H, Maiden M, Kapila A. Sedation practice in the intensive care unit: a UK national survey. Crit Care. 2008;12(6):R152.

39. Happ MB. The power and importance of accommodation for communication impairment in the intensive care unit. Ann Am Thorac Soc. 2016;13(8):1215–6.
40. Radtke JV, Tate JA, Happ MB. Nurses' perceptions of communication training in the ICU. Intensive Crit Care Nurs. 2012;28(1):16–25.
41. Faculty of Intensive Care Medicine, Intensive Care Society. Guidelines for the Provision of Intensive Care Services (GPICS) Edition 2. 2019. https://www.ficm.ac.uk/sites/default/files/gpics-v2.pdf.
42. Rose L, Cook A, Onwumere J, Terblanche E, Pattison N, Metaxa V, et al. Psychological distress and morbidity of family members experiencing virtual visiting in intensive care during COVID-19: an observational cohort study. Intensive Care Med. 2022;48(9):1156–64.
43. Jesus L, Simões J, Voegeli D. Verbal communication with unconscious patients. Acta Paulista de Enfermagem. 2013;26:506–13.
44. Wallace S, McGowan S, Sutt A-L. Benefits and options for voice restoration in mechanically ventilated intensive care unit patients with a tracheostomy. J Intensive Care Soc. 2023;24(1):104–11.
45. Patak L, Gawlinski A, Fung NI, Doering L, Berg J, Henneman EA. Communication boards in critical care: patients' views. Appl Nurs Res. 2006;19(4):182–90.
46. Otuzoglu M, Karahan A. Determining the effectiveness of illustrated communication material for communication with intubated patients at an intensive care unit. Int J Nurs Pract. 2014;20(5):490–8.
47. Kagohara DM, Van Der Meer L, Ramdoss S, O'Reilly MF, Lancioni GE, Davis TN, et al. Using iPods® and iPads® in teaching programs for individuals with developmental disabilities: a systematic review. Res Dev Disabil. 2013;34(1):147–56.
48. Happ MB, Roesch TK, Garrett K. Electronic voice-output communication aids for temporarily nonspeaking patients in a medical intensive care unit: a feasibility study. Heart Lung. 2004;33(2):92–101.
49. Maringelli F, Brienza N, Scorrano F, Grasso F, Gregoretti C. Gaze-controlled, computer-assisted communication in intensive care unit: "speaking through the eyes". Minerva Anestesiol. 2013;79(2):165–75.
50. Sutt AL, Fraser JF. Patients want to be heard-loud and clear! Crit Care. 2017;21(1):6.
51. Prigent H, Orlikowski D, Blumen MB, Leroux K, Legrand L, Lejaille M, et al. Characteristics of tracheostomy phonation valves. Eur Respir J. 2006;27(5):992–6.
52. Sutt AL, Caruana LR, Dunster KR, Cornwell PL, Anstey CM, Fraser JF. Speaking valves in tracheostomised ICU patients weaning off mechanical ventilation—do they facilitate lung recruitment? Crit Care. 2016;20:91.
53. Gross RD, Carrau RL, Slivka WA, Gisser RG, Smith LJ, Zajac DJ, et al. Deglutitive subglottic air pressure and respiratory system recoil. Dysphagia. 2012;27(4):452–9.
54. Gross RD, Mahlmann J, Grayhack JP. Physiologic effects of open and closed tracheostomy tubes on the pharyngeal swallow. Ann Otol Rhinol Laryngol. 2003;112(2):143–52.
55. Wallace S, McGrath BA. Laryngeal complications after tracheal intubation and tracheostomy. BJA Educ. 2021;21(7):250–7.
56. Massery M, Hagins M, Stafford R, Moerchen V, Hodges PW. Effect of airway control by glottal structures on postural stability. J Appl Physiol (1985). 2013;115(4):483–90.
57. Ceron C, Otto D, Signorini AV, Beck MC, Camilis M, Sganzerla D, et al. The effect of speaking valves on ICU mobility of individuals with tracheostomy. Respir Care. 2020;65(2):144–9.
58. Freeman-Sanderson AL, Togher L, Elkins MR, Phipps PR. Return of voice for ventilated tracheostomy patients in ICU: a randomized controlled trial of early-targeted intervention. Crit Care Med. 2016;44(6):1075–81.
59. Sutt AL, Fraser JF. Speaking valves as part of standard care with tracheostomized mechanically ventilated patients in intensive care unit. J Crit Care. 2015;30(5):1119–20.
60. Sutt AL, Cornwell P, Mullany D, Kinneally T, Fraser JF. The use of tracheostomy speaking valves in mechanically ventilated patients results in improved communication and does not prolong ventilation time in cardiothoracic intensive care unit patients. J Crit Care. 2015;30(3):491–4.

61. Heimer J, Eggert S, Fliss B, Meixner E. Fatal bilateral pneumothorax and generalized emphysema following contraindicated speaking-valve application. Forensic Sci Med Pathol. 2019;15(2):239–42.
62. Donzelli J, Brady S, Wesling M, Theisen M. Secretions, occlusion status, and swallowing in patients with a tracheotomy tube: a descriptive study. Ear Nose Throat J. 2006;85(12):831–4.
63. McGrath B, Lynch J, Wilson M, Nicholson L, Wallace S. Above cuff vocalisation: a novel technique for communication in the ventilator-dependent tracheostomy patient. J Intensive Care Soc. 2015;17(1):19–26.

The Intensive Care Unit Environment: Impact and Prevention

9

Lotta Johansson and Deborah Dawson

9.1 Introduction

The advent of intensive care follow-up clinics (Chap. 10) has provided valuable insights into the lived experiences of our patients, both within the ICU and throughout their early recovery. What has become apparent is the multifaceted morbidity of critical illness, with impacts seen on physical, psychological, cognitive and social function. This developing knowledge is having a positive impact on reframing both the patient care we consider appropriate, along with greater consideration of the built environment and the devices we use. Sound and noise from staff conversations and medical equipment has reached an unsustainable level for patients, with the majority of the sound sources placed near the patients' heads, and the alarm volumes set to ensure they can be heard by staff who could be situated anywhere throughout the room or bay. It has been increasingly recognised that the design of the patient room may also impact the patient's circadian rhythm and thus the ability to sleep.

9.2 Sleep and Wakefulness

Sleep is a complex process influenced by many physiological and environmental factors. Lack of sleep is associated with a host of adverse outcomes [1, 2] including stroke, coronary heart disease, diabetes mellitus, metabolic dysregulation, cancer

L. Johansson (✉)
Sahlgrenska University Hospital, University of Gothenburg, Gothenburg, Sweden
e-mail: lotta.k.johansson@vgregion.se; lotta.johansson@fhs.gu.se

D. Dawson
Long Term Ventilation Unit, Royal Hospital for Neurodisability, London, UK
e-mail: ddawson@rhn.org.uk

C. Boulanger, D. McWilliams (eds.), *Passport to Successful Outcomes for Patients Admitted to ICU*, https://doi.org/10.1007/978-3-031-53019-7_9

[3, 4] obesity, stress, decreased immunity, socio-economic status and increased pain sensitivity [3, 5]. Sleep abnormalities, including sleep deprivation, abnormal sleep architecture and sleep disturbance, are common in the intensive care unit [6–9]; these may persist or even develop after the critical illness [1, 10–12] . Recently, concern has been raised that sleep deprivation may impact on delirium in ICU patients and therefore improved sleep may reduce this clinical syndrome and improve ICU morbidity and mortality [13, 14] .

9.2.1   Sleep Architecture and ICU

Normal sleep architecture includes two distinct stages, non-rapid eye movement (NREM) and REM. NREM is comprised of three stages, the first two stages are light sleep and the third, deep slow wave sleep, which is believed to be the most restorative stage of sleep for physiological repair. REM is considered to be necessary for memory consolidation [15, 16]. Studies utilising polysomnography demonstrate that some ICU patients are quantitatively sleep deprived; however more commonly patients are qualitatively deprived, with 40–50% sleep taking place during the day [1, 15–18]. Sleep is fragmented with increased arousals, increased sleep latency, decreased sleep efficiency; most studies suggesting an increase in stages 1 and 2 NREM and a decrease or absence of stage 3 NREM and REM [1, 15–17, 19–22], although one study suggests stage 2 NREM sleep was also decreased [17]. Some patients may suffer poor sleep before admission to an ICU [23], which may continue whilst critically ill; however the majority of patients are likely impacted by the numerous environmental, pathophysiological factors and medication commonly utilised in this care, all of which effect the regulation of sleep [9, 24].

9.2.2   Measuring Sleep

Measuring sleep in the ICU is difficult. The gold standard measure of sleep is polysomnography (PSG), which requires specialist support to apply and interpret accurately [25]. In addition, PSG studies are difficult to interpret in ICU patients due to organ failure, metabolic dysregulation and the medication routinely required to deliver care and treatment [15, 16]. Actigraphy commonly overestimates sleep in ICU patients, as it relies on movement to judge wakefulness [26]. Several survey instruments have been reported to assess patient and/or nurse subjective assessment of sleep; however, the majority lack effective validity and reliability testing [25]. The Richards Campbell Sleep Questionnaire (RCSQ) is utilised widely but requires patients to be awake and cognitively able [27, 28].

9.3   Sound and Noise

9.3.1   Measuring Sound

Sound is generated when a vibration is initiated and sends waves of energy into our ears, creating a sound pressure that can be detected by the ear. Sound is measured objectively in two ways, frequency and amplitude, both are fundamental aspects of how sound is perceived. Sound pressure (amplitude) is measured in Pascals (Pa). The human ear can register more than a million Pa; therefore sound pressure level (SPL) is commonly measured by the logarithmic value decibel (dB). The quietest sound people can hear is 1 dB and sounds above 120 dB cause discomfort and even pain. This logarithmic scale means that a SPL of 3 dB is a doubling of the sound pressure level (50 dB + 50 dB = 53 dB); however, 8–10 dB is double the loudness. The logarithmic scale is often adjusted to take into account the reduced sensitivity of human hearing to high and low frequencies and it is then called dBA or A-weighted decibels [29]. Sound frequency is measured in hertz (Hz); 1 Hz equals one cycle per second. People with normal hearing can typically hear from approximately 50–20,000 Hz (20 KHz). A 50 Hz sound would be similar to a low bass drum and a 20 KHz sound would be a very high frequency, such as a shrill whistle. The hearing threshold varies with frequency, which means that a low frequency sound must be loud (dB) in order to be audible [29]. What is interesting and challenging about sound is that it is both a physiological and subjective experience. The definition of noise is unwanted, uncontrollable or unpredictable sound and additionally signifies a negative subjective response. Whether or not a sound is considered a noise depends on both its acoustic properties and its interference with intended activities.

9.3.2   Sound in the ICU

The World Health Organization (WHO) guidelines are the most frequently quoted guidance and suggest hospital noise levels should average 35 dBA during the day and 30 dBA at night [30]. Several authors have suggested these levels are unachievable [31, 32], as sound measured in an empty patient room is commonly reported to be equal to or greater than 35 dBA [31, 32] and evidence suggests that during the day, average SPL range between 52.5 dBA [33] and 64.8 dBA [34]. It is hard to give one unanimous picture of the acoustic environment in the ICU, as this is influenced by numerous factors, such as building layouts, the numbers of beds and staffing. The complexity of the soundscape in the ICU area may however be described from three different perspectives, firstly from an acoustic perspective, i.e. a description of the high SPL and the wide variation in sound frequencies. This research has found that the SPLs in patient rooms in the ICU generally exceed existing international and national guidelines [30–38] with most high levels of noise originating from a few specific areas, such as the nursing station or the area very close to the patients' head [39]. The frequency ranges of alarms (2.5–3.15 KHz) are similar to both a human scream and a baby's cry [39]. Single-patient rooms are rare in many countries, which means that seriously ill patients often become the audience to other patients' alarms and activities. This means that the critically ill patient is exposed to very high SPL sequences 24 h a day [31, 40].

Secondly, we can investigate sound in terms of the large number of sound sources [41, 42]. Of these sources, medical and nursing interventions, alarms from mechanical ventilators and staff speech have been found to be the most dominant and impactful noise sources [32, 38, 42, 43], generating up to 75 dB [44, 45] and 10% of the total episodes of noise [32]. Other examples of sound sources are ringing telephones, change of dialysate bags and the pneumatic pumps driving the mattress [32, 41]. The different sounds come unexpectedly and suddenly [46] which increases the likelihood of arousal and sleep disturbances [42]. What this means physiologically for the patient is not clear, but it likely does not favour recovery.

Lastly, the soundscape can be described from the perspective of the critically ill patient. Contrary to what many believe, despite their fatigue and critical illness, most patients receiving care in the ICU hear and are aware of the ambient sounds during their stay [9, 40, 46, 47]. It is also important to note that fewer sedative drugs are used today in the ICU, which means the patients are more likely to be awake and conscious, making them even more susceptible to noise. Approximately half of patients recalled the surrounding noise as disturbing or stressful [48, 49] and many patients have also characterised ICU sound as noise [46], with much of this sound ingression from agitated patients or treatment to patients cared for in the same room or bay [40, 50, 51]. Extremely disturbing and constantly loud were the words patients themselves used in qualitative research [9, 47]. Not all sound is described as problematic and the context of the sound appears to be an important factor. Patients describe nurse and family voices as reassuring [51] or sound as soothing and pleasing and in some cases, sound gave hope, support and helped orient the patient in terms of time and space [46]. It seems that the sound environment of the ICU is acceptable to patients when it is deemed necessary, but similar sounds may be described as frightening or annoying if they are considered unnecessary [32]. This complex sound environment then means that one measure is insufficient to make improvement and the noise problem requires more than one solution.

9.3.3   The Impact of Noise on the ICU Patient

It is well-established that noise adversely affects sleep and health in healthy individuals [52].

Noise can activate autonomic and neuroendocrine systems, resulting in increased cardiac output and blood pressure, decreased digestive secretion, increased metabolism and increased respiratory rate [52, 53]. Noise and its physical impact on patients with critical illnesses are, however, more difficult to clarify because there are many other aspects that seem to affect the individuals' medical condition in relation to critical illness, such as infections and drugs. For example, opioids decrease stage NREM3 sleep and, at higher doses, also decrease REM sleep [54].

Sleep and confusion are the two most studied areas when it comes to sound and its impact on patients with critical illnesses. Critically ill patients sleep poorly during their time in the ICU and noise is one of the factors that disrupts their sleep cycle [36, 42, 55]. However, the relationship between noise and sleep is not entirely clear and therefore, the importance of noise and its impact on sleep for in the critically ill is debated [56]. For instance, there is a discrepancy between self-reported sleep quality and the biophysiological data that are obtained during sleep. Patients themselves describe in interviews sudden arousals and awakenings because of voices in their rooms [57–59] while other studies that utilise objective sleep measures have reported conflicting results [56, 60]. One study found that 60% of awakenings are triggered by a noise higher than 77 dB [42].The suggestion is that sound and noise are factors that affect sleep, but we do not know precisely how and to what extent.

Restorative periods were first described by Ryherd and colleagues [61] who noted that there were periods of time when the background noise was quieter and foreground sound less fluctuant, thus perhaps providing time for rest. These periods were more common at night but were described as restorative if they occurred at any time of the day or night. Other authors [62, 63] have also attempted to define these periods, describing longer cumulative restorative time in single rooms [63] and referring back to earlier study utilising polysomnography [17] to define restorative periods relative to background noise [62]. Currently, restorative periods as described are thought to be insufficient to improve the patient's wellbeing or quality of sleep, since the intervals between sound events were too short to enable restorative sleep [61, 62].

ICU delirium is a multifaceted disorder that has been discussed in relation to high SPLs and complex sound environments in intensive care. Since the cause of the onset of ICU delirium is not yet clear and no cure exists, one line of research has focused on how to prevent the condition. As a part of this, a few intervention studies have investigated how noise-reducing measures such as having single-bed rooms [63], using earplugs at night [64] and developing sound-reduction protocols [65] affect the development of confusion and ICU delirium. The results indicate that there is a connection between noise and ICU delirium, and that noise reduction measures might prevent its development. On the other hand, a larger study (the UNDERPIN-ICU study) [66], conducted in ICUs of ten centres, and which aims was to reduce delirium using a multicomponent programme including noise reduction, found no significant increase in the number of delirium-free days. Currently more studies are needed in this area. More research is also needed to clarify whether the effect is indirect (i.e. whether it is the improved sleep that prevents the development of ICU delirium and confusion) or if the decreased development of ICU delirium is a direct response to reduced sound levels. In summary, sound and noise are factors that in some way influence sleep and the development of confusion in critically ill patients. Therefore, it is reasonable to surmise that an improvement in the sound environment in the ICU would also increase the probability of a faster recovery for a vulnerable and fragile patient group.

9.4   Light and Dark

9.4.1   Measuring Light Intensity

Light energy is a form of electromagnetic radiation, which travels in waves and is the only energy visible to the human eye. Light energy is measured in nanometres (nm) and as for sound its frequency is measured in hertz (Hz). Humans can sense light energy for wavelengths between 400 and 700 nm and turn it into images. The eye is sensitive to a very wide range of light intensity but at low levels loses the ability to identify detail and working under poor lighting causes fatigue. Light intensity or illuminance is measured in lux (lx). Outdoor day-time light levels vary according to the weather and the time of the day and year, however range from approximately 1000 to 120,000 lx, with night-time levels below 1 lx. Light levels measured in an ICU also vary dependant on the provision of both natural and artificial lighting, time of day and orientation of the room. One study suggests that day-time measures range between 3 and 1812 lx, with night-time levels between 1 and 1306 lx [67]; however many other studies do not record as broad a range with a general trend to day-time levels being extremely poor and artificial light levels increased at night [33, 68, 69].

9.4.2   Circadian Rhythms

Sleep and wakefulness are regulated by the circadian rhythm for wakefulness and homeostatic sleep processes for sleep [70]. Light is the most important zeitgeber, a rhythmically occurring natural phenomenon which acts as a cue in the regulation of the body's circadian rhythm. Circadian rhythms respond primarily to light and darkness to modulate physiological, biochemical and behavioural processes, which means that proper light is of importance [33, 71, 72]. In the ICU patient, the normal rhythmic profiles of blood pressure, heart rate, temperature, motor activity and the level of cortisol and melatonin are altered [70], and many of these processes are affected by the use of sedation [1]. Later studies have found that disturbance of the circadian rhythm of melatonin and cortisol secretion may be associated with the development of delirium in ICU patients [73, 74].

9.4.3   Light Intensity in the ICU

The study of light intensity in ICU is less common than that for sound [75] but, more and more studies are being conducted in the area. It is known that the average daytime light levels in both the ICU and non-ICU environment are low [33, 68, 76, 77]. Furthermore, peak light levels seems to occur later in the day instead of in the morning [76] which means that the lightning in the patient rooms are insufficient to promote normal circadian entrainment. The lighting at night seems to be relatively dim but slightly higher than at home, as one patient describes; *it was not completely dark but more like twilight* [78]. Interruptions often occur for brief sequences with bright light [79]. About one third of the patients in the ICU report that night-time light is disruptive to their sleep [80]. A recent study also found that lighting in the ICU patient room may have impact on the critically ill patients' physiological parameters such as heart rate [81].

Studies in the area [33, 68, 76, 77] highlight a wide variety of reported light levels which appear to be dependent on the time of the day the study was completed, the orientation of the room and the availability of natural and artificial light, but also the cultural behaviours of staff. There is some evidence to suggest that if lighting was optimised during the day, both by improving the built environment and by the actions of staff caring for critically ill patients, circadian rhythms may be less impacted. Two reports describe a trial of cycled lighting in an ICU patient room [78, 82]. The first discusses the patient perspective of light and use of cycled lighting [78]. The cycled lighting system simulated natural light providing 14 different lighting levels over a 24 h period, lux levels varied from 2 lx (night-time 21.30–07.00 h) and 615 lx at 08.00–10.00 h. One hundred patients cared for either in this modified room ($n = 48$) or an alternative without cycled lighting ($n = 52$) were surveyed to understand their perception of the light environment. A significant number of patients favoured the lighting environment in the intervention room. Patients who had experienced the cycled lighting were interviewed ($n = 19$); this suggested they found the lighting pleasant and that it engendered feelings of calm and security, although it did not appear to impact reports of improved sleep. The second report [82] describes the results of a pilot study comparing the circadian rhythms of patients in the cycled lighting room with a normal patient room during their last 24 h in the ICU. This demonstrated evidence of a circadian cycle which was not improved by the cycled lighting. This may have been due to the patient being at the end of their ICU stay when the circadian rhythm may have been improved or that the study underpowered to demonstrate a difference.

It is clear that before we can understand the impact light has on circadian rhythms, sleep, delirium and the outcome of the critically ill patient, there is a need for more and larger studies into the management of light intensity.

9.5   Humanising the ICU Environment

9.5.1   Improving Sleep in the ICU

Despite many years of study describing sleep abnormalities in ICU, few units have changed practice [83, 84]. ICU staff recognise both the importance of sleep and the presence of sleep disruption during an ICU stay; however, routine use of objective tools to measure sleep and the use of sleep bundles/protocols is infrequent [83, 84] although sleep assessment appears to be more common in units where nurses influence sleep strategies [84]. There is also considerable variation in interventions to promote sleep across countries, including noise reduction, dimming lights, reducing nurse interventions, keeping patients awake during the day and, given the ease of use it is surprising that few units use ear plugs or reduce alarm volumes [84]. Despite this, earplugs and eye masks have been shown to improve sleep quality and quantity in healthy subjects exposed to ICU noise and light suggesting they may be useful in ICU patients [85–87]. Furthermore, earplugs have been shown to reduce or delay symptoms of delirium or confusion [85].

9.5.2   What Can We Do to Prevent a Noisy Environment?

Many studies have measured the impact of programmes to reduce noise at night and improve sleep in the ICU with generally disappointing results. Several studies have demonstrated statistically significant improvements in noise levels at night following the implementation of a night time sound reduction protocol; however the level of reduction was clinically and acoustically irrelevant and did not improve patient reported quality of sleep [88–92]. The sound environment can however easily be influenced, and therefore we should do everything we can to reduce sound levels in the patients' rooms to improve patient comfort and the potential for sleep during critical illness. First of all, all staff working with and around the patient, including management, must be aware of the sound/noise they make and its potential impact on the patient. We know that ICU staff have poor knowledge when it comes to noise and its health effects [93, 94]. Secondly, we need to clarify to the patients that the staff have control over the technical equipment and its alarms. It is important to explain continuously to the patient what the vital sounds mean, where they come from and why they are necessary. Third, there is a great need for patient involvement. We need to help the patients to take control of their sound environment by offering, for example, access to earplugs or earmuffs and/or the possibility of quiet time. More specifically, there are a lot of aspects caregivers can do to reduce the noise in the ICU patient room, see Table 9.1.

9.5.3   What Can We Do to Ensure Appropriate Light Intensity?

Despite critically ill patients' eyelids frequently being closed in the ICU, it is important to attempt to retain/re-establish a circadian rhythm for these patients, which in turn may improve both sleep and reduce the incidence of delirium. For example, a recent study found that a circadian light system had positive impact on ICU patients durations of deep sleep, light sleep and total sleep [107]. However, a number of factors affect the circadian rhythm in patients in the ICU such as noise [32, 35], feeding [108, 109], medication [110] and patient care interactions [111]. This means that there is a lot we can do to improve the circadian rhythm of the patients the ICU. Although more study is required, it would seem reasonable to utilise all available light during the day, by opening blinds and using artificial light to its full capacity. Additionally, early work studying bright light therapy may provide an alternative method of restoring circadian rhythms for ICU patients [112, 113]. As for sound, it is important that staff are made aware of the impact of inappropriate lighting use,

Table 9.1 This table summarises a number of different actions, divided in three categories, that can be taken to improve the sound environment in the ICU patient room [36, 63, 65, 95–106]

Simple measures for the individual caregiver	Measures that need collaboration	Complex and/or expensive measures
Adjusting the alarm settings to patient need	Reminding each other (verbally or in writing) about attenuating sounds	Noise-cancelling headphones
Lower the sound levels of the alarms	Having scheduled quiet times	Sound absorbing panels
Coordinate care activities	Implementing sound-reduction protocols	Non-acoustic alarms
Handle the materials and equipment carefully	Not placing a newly arrived, acutely ill patient next to a patient with major need for sleep	Improvement of the physical space
Distribute earplugs	Educational arrangements concerning sound and its effects	Improvement of the technical design
Speak more quietly	Education on the use of technical equipment to promote unnecessary sounds	Single patient rooms
Keep doors closed	Involved management	
Lowering the bed rail gently	Managing alarms limits against risk profiles	
Preparing drugs, trollies and opening intravenous packaging away from the bed space		
Avoid taking mobile phone calls at the bed space		

and therefore utilise lighting and darkness effectively for patient care, but have sufficient work station light so as not to impact their health. In the future, we should expect that units will be designed to fully appreciate the impact of the built environment on patient welfare and outcome. This would include building bright, light rooms, with the equivalent of blackout blinds for night time use. The lighting of an intensive care unit should also require careful consideration to ensure lighting for emergency procedures, lighting for day time and also lower level lighting for nighttime use; it is possible this will include cycled lighting. The light should be positioned to achieve a balance to ensure staff have appropriate work lighting, but patients are not disturbed by this.

9.5.4 Other Strategies to Improve and Humanise the ICU Environment

So far, this chapter has concentrated on areas where there is a reasonable body of evidence to improve the sound environment and also to some extent the lighting for the intensive care patient. There are however many other aspects of practice that can be improved or accented to humanise the intensive care unit environment and utilise more appropriately sensory stimuli such as hearing, sight, touch and smell. A recent systematic review, as with many analyses of a large number of heterogenous interventions and patient populations, suggests little effectiveness for non-pharmacological interventions in reducing delirium [114]. This report does however highlight a range of interventions that in themselves are unlikely to do harm and may be of benefit to critically ill patients [114]. Much of this practice is congruent with the principles of Family Centred Care, which today should be core to the care of patients admitted to the ICU [115]. One of these principles is to enable family presence, but also provide support to those families in the ICU. Visiting should not be restricted and support should be in place to ensure children may visit if they and the patient wish this, but in doing so the children should receive age related support pre and post visit [116]. An innovative but simple pilot study tested the effect of an automated reorientation intervention where a recorded family member's voice was played during the daytime and demonstrated an improvement in delirium free days in the intervention group [117]. This provided the patient with regular reassurance of where they were and that they were being cared for utilising a family members voice, but without the need for families to be present at all times, something that many families find difficult when trying to maintain the social reality of family life. Diaries are now common for longer term patients which may assist with orientation, knowing the patient as a person and giving them back social control [118–120]. An extension of this idea is pet therapy or animal assisted intervention, which appears to be growing in popularity. It is thought that this introducing pets and animals into the ICU environment may reduce suffering, increase engagement and reduce physiological burden [121] and it will certainly humanise the environment. Several authors provide guidance as to how this be achieved in an acute hospital [108]. However, infection control, welfare of the pet, assessment of patient suitability for pet therapy, religious and cultural issues related to pets, consideration of staff fears about pets or allergies to animals need are areas to be discussed in the future before implementation. Music is frequently played in an ICU, but often not necessarily focused on the patient's preferences or wellbeing. Several studies have highlighted the benefit of music therapy in reducing sedation and anxiety [122–124], in patients receiving ventilatory support for acute respiratory failure, self-initiated music resulted in a reduction in anxiety and sedation intensity compared with usual care [122] and may reduce weaning times [123].

In summary, the environment and context in which we care for our fragile and vulnerable critically ill patients is as important as the physical treatment we traditionally provide. Sleep is illusive and delirium common in the ICU; however through sound and light research, we are starting to understand how we might be able to improve both the environment, for staff and patients, but also the outcomes for our patients. If we are to improve the patients' condition, everyone who works in intensive care must contribute to appropriate sound reduction measures, improve lighting and establish a relationship with our patients and their families to humanise the environment. However, it is also equally important that professionals take responsibility for the sound and light environment being included in strategic planning, when purchasing medical technical equipment and when building or rebuilding premises.

Key Take Home Messages

- Sleep abnormalities are common in the intensive care unit; these may persist or even develop after the critical illness.
- Measuring sleep quality and quantity is complex in the critically ill patient.
- Sleep bundles or interventions to promote sleep are inconsistent and infrequently utilised across countries.
- The soundscape of an ICU may be described by noise levels, sources of sound and from the patient perspective.
- Multiple studies have identified that sound pressure levels in the ICU exceed the current WHO guidance and that patients recall noise in ICU as disturbing or stressful.
- Light levels impact the regulation of the circadian rhythm and in ICU are commonly found to be too low during the day and too high at night.
- The relationship between noise, light levels, sleep and delirium in the ICU patient is not clear; it is however likely that environmental factors such as inappropriate poor lighting and noise will have a negative impact.
- There are some promising interventions that may improve the patient environment including better utilisation of natural and artificial lighting, noise cancelling headphones, improvement of the built environment for both light and noise, ensuring strategies to prevent or reduce delirium and applying the principles of Family Centred Care.

References

1. Pisani MA, et al. Sleep in the intensive care unit. Am J Respir Crit Care Med. 2015;191(7):731–8.
2. Liew SC, Aung T. Sleep deprivation and its association with diseases—a review. Sleep Med. 2021;77:192–204.
3. Grandner MA, et al. Mortality associated with short sleep duration: the evidence, the possible mechanisms, and the future. Sleep Med Rev. 2010;14(3):191–203.
4. Yin J, et al. Relationship of sleep duration with all-cause mortality and cardiovascular events: a systematic review and dose-response meta-analysis of prospective cohort studies. J Am Heart Assoc. 2017;6(9):e005947.
5. Schrimpf M, et al. The effect of sleep deprivation on pain perception in healthy subjects: a meta-analysis. Sleep Med. 2015;16(11):1313–20.
6. Tembo AC, Parker V. Factors that impact on sleep in intensive care patients. Intensive Crit Care Nurs. 2009;25(6):314–22.
7. Prajapat B, et al. Evaluation of sleep architecture using 24-hour polysomnography in patients recovering from critical illness in an intensive care unit and high dependency unit: a longitudinal, prospective, and observational study. J Crit Care Med. 2021;7(4):257–66.
8. Telias I, Wilcox ME. Sleep and circadian rhythm in critical illness. Crit Care. 2019;23(1):82.
9. Lewandowska K, et al. Sleep deprivation from the perspective of a patient hospitalized in the intensive care unit-qualitative study. Healthcare (Basel). 2020;8(3):351.
10. McKinley S, et al. Health-related quality of life and associated factors in intensive care unit survivors 6 months after discharge. Am J Crit Care. 2016;25(1):52–8.

11. Wilcox ME, et al. Actigraphic measures of sleep on the wards after ICU discharge. J Crit Care. 2019;54:163–9.
12. Edmiston EA, Hardin HK, Dolansky MA. Sleep quality in the advanced heart failure ICU. Clin Nurs Res. 2023;32(4):691–8.
13. Weinhouse GL, et al. Bench-to-bedside review: delirium in ICU patients—importance of sleep deprivation. Crit Care. 2009;13(6):234.
14. Daou M, et al. Abnormal sleep, circadian rhythm disruption, and delirium in the ICU: are they related? Front Neurol. 2020;11:549908.
15. Hardin KA. Sleep in the ICU potential mechanisms and clinical implications. Chest. 2009;136(1):284–94.
16. Kamdar BB, Needham DM, Collop NA. Sleep deprivation in critical illness: its role in physical and psychological recovery. J Intensive Care Med. 2012;27(2):97–111.
17. Freedman NS, et al. Abnormal sleep/wake cycles and the effect of environmental noise on sleep disruption in the intensive care unit. Am J Respir Crit Care Med. 2001;163(2):451–7.
18. Fanfulla F, et al. Sleep disturbances in patients admitted to a step-down unit after ICU discharge: the role of mechanical ventilation. Sleep. 2011;34(3):355–62.
19. Gabor JY, et al. Contribution of the intensive care unit environment to sleep disruption in mechanically ventilated patients and healthy subjects. Am J Respir Crit Care Med. 2003;167(5):708–15.
20. Elliott R, et al. Characterisation of sleep in intensive care using 24-hour polysomnography: an observational study. Crit Care. 2013;17(2):R46.
21. Fowler SB, et al. Sleep in aneurysmal subarachnoid hemorrhage patients during critical and acute care. Dimens Crit Care Nurs. 2021;40(2):118–24.
22. Boyko Y, Jennum P, Toft P. Sleep quality and circadian rhythm disruption in the intensive care unit: a review. Nat Sci Sleep. 2017;9:277–84.
23. Little A, et al. A patient survey of sleep quality in the intensive care unit. Minerva Anestesiol. 2012;78(4):406–14.
24. Gehlbach BK, et al. Temporal disorganization of circadian rhythmicity and sleep-wake regulation in mechanically ventilated patients receiving continuous intravenous sedation. Sleep. 2012;35(8):1105–14.
25. Jeffs EL, Darbyshire JL. Measuring sleep in the intensive care unit: a critical appraisal of the use of subjective methods. J Intensive Care Med. 2019;34(9):751–60.
26. Schwab K, et al. Use of actigraphy to evaluate sleep in the ICU: a systematic review. Chest. 2016;150(4):217A.
27. Ritmala-Castren M, et al. Investigating the construct and concurrent validity of the Richards-Campbell Sleep Questionnaire with intensive care unit patients and home sleepers. Aust Crit Care. 2022;35(2):130–5.
28. Alsulami G, Rice AM, Kidd L. Prospective repeated assessment of self-reported sleep quality and sleep disruptive factors in the intensive care unit: acceptability of daily assessment of sleep quality. BMJ Open. 2019;9(6):e029957.
29. Speaks CE. Introduction to sound: acoustics for the hearing and speech sciences. San Diego, CA: Singular Publishing Group; 1999.
30. Berglund B, et al. Guidelines for community noise. Geneva: World Health Organization; 1999.
31. Darbyshire JL, Young JD. An investigation of sound levels on intensive care units with reference to the WHO guidelines. Crit Care. 2013;17(5):R187.
32. Dawson D, et al. Towards the acoustical characterisation of an intensive care unit. In: Proceedings of the Institute of Acoustics, vol. 40, part 1; 2018.
33. Danielson SJ, et al. Looking for light in the din: an examination of the circadian-disrupting properties of a medical intensive care unit. Intensive Crit Care Nurs. 2018;46:57–63.
34. Memoli G, et al. Towards the acoustical characterisation of an intensive care unit. Appl Acoust. 2014;79:124–30.
35. Johansson L. Being critically ill and surrounded by sound and noise. Patient experiences, staff awareness and future challenges; 2014.

36. Simons KS, et al. Noise in the intensive care unit and its influence on sleep quality: a multi-center observational study in Dutch intensive care units. Crit Care. 2018;22(1):250.
37. Naef AC, et al. Methods for measuring and identifying sounds in the intensive care unit. Front Med. 2022;9:836203.
38. Lucchini A, et al. Sound and light levels in a general intensive care unit without windows to provide natural light. Dimens Crit Care Nurs. 2023;42(2):115–23.
39. Darbyshire JL, et al. Mapping sources of noise in an intensive care unit. Anaesthesia. 2019;74(8):1018–25.
40. Johansson L, et al. The sound environment in an ICU patient room—a content analysis of sound levels and patient experiences. Intensive Crit Care Nurs. 2012;28(5):269–79.
41. Czempik PF, et al. Impact of sound levels and patient-related factors on sleep of patients in the intensive care unit: a cross-sectional cohort study. Sci Rep. 2020;10(1):19207.
42. Elbaz M, et al. Sound level intensity severely disrupts sleep in ventilated ICU patients throughout a 24-h period: a preliminary 24-h study of sleep stages and associated sound levels. Ann Intensive Care. 2017;7(1):25.
43. Choiniere DB. The effects of hospital noise. Nurs Adm Q. 2010;34(4):327–33.
44. Akansel N, Kaymakci S. Effects of intensive care unit noise on patients: a study on coronary artery bypass graft surgery patients. J Clin Nurs. 2008;17(12):1581–90.
45. Tsiou C, et al. Noise sources and levels in the Evgenidion Hospital intensive care unit. Intensive Care Med. 1998;24(8):845–7.
46. Johansson L, Bergbom I, Lindahl B. Meanings of being critically ill in a sound-intensive ICU patient room—a phenomenological hermeneutical study. Open Nurs J. 2012;6(1):108–16.
47. Tronstad O, et al. Doing time in an Australian ICU the experience and environment from the perspective of patients and family members. Aust Crit Care. 2021;34(3):254–62.
48. Hofhuis JG, et al. Experiences of critically ill patients in the ICU. Intensive Crit Care Nurs. 2008;24(5):300–13.
49. Rose L, et al. Psychological wellbeing, health related quality of life and memories of intensive care and a specialised weaning centre reported by survivors of prolonged mechanical ventilation. Intensive Crit Care Nurs. 2014;30(3):145–51.
50. Samuelson K, Lundberg D, Fridlund B. Memory in relation to depth of sedation in adult mechanically ventilated intensive care patients. Intensive Care Med. 2006;32(5):660–7.
51. Dawson D, et al. Patient, visitor and staff perception of noise in an intensive care unit in BACCN conference 2019: Edinburgh.
52. WHO, NIGHT NOISE GUIDELINES (NNGL) FOR EUROPE Final implementation report. 2007. https://ec.europa.eu/health/ph_projects/2003/action3/docs/2003_08_frep_en.pdf.
53. Hsu T, et al. Noise pollution in hospitals: impact on patients. J Clin Outcomes Manag. 2012;19(7):301–9.
54. Schweitzer PK, Randazzo AC. Chapter 45—Drugs that disturb sleep and wakefulness. In: Kryger M, Roth T, Dement WC, editors. Principles and practice of sleep medicine (sixth edition). Amsterdam: Elsevier; 2017. p. 480–498.e8.
55. Persson Waye K, et al. Improvement of intensive care unit sound environment and analyses of consequences on sleep: an experimental study. Sleep Med. 2013;14(12):1334–40.
56. Horsten S, et al. Systematic review of the effects of intensive-care-unit noise on sleep of healthy subjects and the critically ill. Br J Anaesth. 2018;120(3):443–52.
57. Karlsson V, Lindahl B, Bergbom I. Patients' statements and experiences concerning receiving mechanical ventilation: a prospective video-recorded study. Nurs Inq. 2012;19(3):247–58.
58. McKinley S, et al. Vulnerability and security in seriously ill patients in intensive care. Intensive Crit Care Nurs. 2002;18(1):27–36.
59. Samuelson KAM. Unpleasant and pleasant memories of intensive care in adult mechanically ventilated patients—findings from 250 interviews. Intensive Crit Care Nurs. 2011;27(2):76–84.
60. Xie H, Kang J, Mills GH. Clinical review: the impact of noise on patients' sleep and the effectiveness of noise reduction strategies in intensive care units. Crit Care. 2009;13(2):208.

61. Ryherd EE, Waye KP, Ljungkvist L. Characterizing noise and perceived work environment in a neurological intensive care unit. J Acoust Soc Am. 2008;123(2):747–56.
62. Park MH, et al. Analysis of the soundscape in an intensive care unit based on the annotation of an audio recording. J Acoust Soc Am. 2014;135(4):1875–86.
63. Tegnestedt C, et al. Levels and sources of sound in the intensive care unit—an observational study of three room types. Acta Anaesthesiol Scand. 2013;57(8):1041–50.
64. Van Rompaey B, et al. The effect of earplugs during the night on the onset of delirium and sleep perception: a randomized controlled trial in intensive care patients. Crit Care. 2012;16(3):R73.
65. van de Pol I, van Iterson M, Maaskant J. Effect of nocturnal sound reduction on the incidence of delirium in intensive care unit patients: an interrupted time series analysis. Intensive Crit Care Nurs. 2017;41:18–25.
66. Rood PJT, et al. The impact of nursing delirium preventive interventions in the ICU: a multicenter cluster-randomized controlled clinical trial. Am J Respir Crit Care Med. 2021;204(6):682–91.
67. Voigt LP, et al. Monitoring sound and light continuously in an intensive care unit patient room: a pilot study. J Crit Care. 2017;39:36–9.
68. Fan EP, et al. Abnormal environmental light exposure in the intensive care environment. J Crit Care. 2017;40:11–4.
69. Verceles AC, et al. Ambient light levels and critical care outcomes. J Crit Care. 2013;28(1):110.e1–8.
70. Felten M, et al. Circadian rhythm disruption in critically ill patients. Acta Physiol. 2023;238(1):e13962.
71. Chiu W-C, et al. The impact of windows on the outcomes of medical intensive care unit patients. Int J Gerontol. 2018;12(1):67–70.
72. Lee HJ, et al. Association of natural light exposure and delirium according to the presence or absence of windows in the intensive care unit. Acute Crit Care. 2021;36(4):332–41.
73. Li J, et al. Circadian rhythm disturbance and delirium in ICU patients: a prospective cohort study. BMC Anesthesiol. 2023;23(1):1–203.
74. Sun T, et al. Sleep and circadian rhythm disturbances in intensive care unit (ICU)-acquired delirium: a case–control study. J Int Med Res. 2021;49(3):300060521990502.
75. Lindskov FO, Iversen HK, West AS. Clinical outcomes of light therapy in hospitalized patients—a systematic review. Chronobiol Int. 2022;39(2):299–310.
76. Jaiswal SJ, Garcia S, Owens RL. Sound and light levels are similarly disruptive in ICU and non-ICU wards. J Hosp Med. 2017;12(10):798–804.
77. Lusczek ER, Knauert MP. Light levels in ICU patient rooms: dimming of daytime light in occupied rooms. J Patient Exp. 2021;8:23743735211033104.
78. Engwall M, et al. Lighting, sleep and circadian rhythm: an intervention study in the intensive care unit. Intensive Crit Care Nurs. 2015;31(6):325–35.
79. Merilainen M, Kyngas H, Ala-Kokko T. 24-Hour intensive care: an observational study of an environment and events. Intensive Crit Care Nurs. 2010;26(5):246–53.
80. Honarmand K, et al. A systematic review of risk factors for sleep disruption in critically ill adults. Crit Care Med. 2020;48(7):1066–74.
81. Korompeli A, et al. Circadian disruption of ICU patients: a review of pathways, expression and interventions. J Crit Care. 2017;38:269–77.
82. Engwall M, et al. The effect of cycled lighting in the intensive care unit on sleep, activity and physiological parameters: a pilot study. Intensive Crit Care Nurs. 2017;41:26–32.
83. Kamdar BB, et al. Perceptions and practices regarding sleep in the intensive care unit. A survey of 1,223 critical care providers. Ann Am Thorac Soc. 2016;13(8):1370–7.
84. Hofhuis JGM, et al. Clinical practices to promote sleep in the ICU: a multinational survey. Int J Nurs Stud. 2018;81:107–14.
85. Litton E, et al. The efficacy of earplugs as a sleep hygiene strategy for reducing delirium in the ICU: a systematic review and meta-analysis. Crit Care Med. 2016;44(5):992–9.

86. Obanor OO, et al. The impact of earplugs and eye masks on sleep quality in surgical ICU patients at risk for frequent awakenings. Crit Care Med. 2021;49(9):E822–32.
87. Fang CS, et al. Effect of earplugs and eye masks on the sleep quality of intensive care unit patients: a systematic review and meta-analysis. J Adv Nurs. 2021;77(11):4321–31.
88. Tainter CR, et al. Noise levels in surgical ICUs are consistently above recommended standards. Crit Care Med. 2016;44(1):147–52.
89. Plummer NR, et al. SoundEar noise warning devices cause a sustained reduction in ambient noise in adult critical care. J Intensive Care Soc. 2019;20(2):106–10.
90. Guisasola-Rabes M, et al. Effectiveness of a visual noise warning system on noise levels in a surgical ICU: a quality improvement programme. Eur J Anaesthesiol. 2019;36(11):857–62.
91. Walder B, et al. Effects of guidelines implementation in a surgical intensive care unit to control nighttime light and noise levels. Crit Care Med. 2000;28(7):2242–7.
92. Monsen MG, Edéll-Gustafsson UM. Noise and sleep disturbance factors before and after implementation of a behavioural modification programme. Intensive Crit Care Nurs. 2005;21(4):208–19.
93. Johansson L, et al. Noise in the ICU patient room—staff knowledge and clinical improvements. Intensive Crit Care Nurs. 2016;35(35):1–9.
94. Christensen M. What knowledge do ICU nurses have with regard to the effects of noise exposure in the intensive care unit? Intensive Crit Care Nurs. 2005;21(4):199–207.
95. Dube JA, et al. Environmental noise sources and interventions to minimize them: a tale of 2 hospitals. J Nurs Care Qual. 2008;23(3):216–24; quiz 225–6.
96. Lawson N, et al. Sound intensity and noise evaluation in a critical care unit. Am J Crit Care. 2010;19(6):e88–98.
97. Scotto CJ, et al. Earplugs improve patients' subjective experience of sleep in critical care. Nurs Crit Care. 2009;14(4):180–4.
98. Hu R-F, et al. Effects of earplugs and eye masks combined with relaxing music on sleep, melatonin and cortisol levels in ICU patients: a randomized controlled trial. Crit Care. 2015;19(1):115.
99. Jones C, Dawson D. Eye masks and earplugs improve patient's perception of sleep. Nurs Crit Care. 2012;17(5):247–54.
100. Czaplik M, et al. Psychoacoustic analysis of noise and the application of earplugs in an ICU: a randomised controlled clinical trial. Eur J Anaesthesiol. 2016;33(1):14–21.
101. Dennis CM, et al. Benefits of quiet time for neuro-intensive care patients. J Neurosci Nurs. 2010;42(4):217–24.
102. Patel J, et al. The effect of a multicomponent multidisciplinary bundle of interventions on sleep and delirium in medical and surgical intensive care patients. Anaesthesia. 2014;69(6):540–9.
103. Gallacher S, et al. An experimental model to measure the ability of headphones with active noise control to reduce patient's exposure to noise in an intensive care unit. Intensive Care Med Exp. 2017;5(1):47.
104. Farrehi PM, Nallamothu BK, Navvab M. Reducing hospital noise with sound acoustic panels and diffusion: a controlled study. BMJ Qual Saf. 2016;25(8):644–6.
105. Jousselme C, et al. Efficacy and mode of action of a noise-sensor light alarm to decrease noise in the pediatric intensive care unit: a prospective, randomized study. Pediatr Crit Care Med. 2011;12(2):e69–72.
106. Luetz A, et al. Feasibility of noise reduction by a modification in ICU environment. Physiol Meas. 2016;37(7):1041–55.
107. Pamuk K, Turan N. The effect of light on sleep quality and physiological parameters in patients in the intensive care unit. Appl Nurs Res. 2022;66:151607.
108. Abbott SM, Malkani RG, Zee PC. Circadian disruption and human health: a bidirectional relationship. Eur J Neurosci. 2020;51(1):567–83.
109. Kouw IWK, Heilbronn LK, Van Zanten ARH. Intermittent feeding and circadian rhythm in critical illness. Curr Opin Crit Care. 2022;28(4):381–8.
110. Mundigler G, et al. Impaired circadian rhythm of melatonin secretion in sedated critically ill patients with severe sepsis. Crit Care Med. 2002;30(3):536–40.

111. Ritmala-Castren M, et al. Sleep and nursing care activities in an intensive care unit: ICU patients' sleep and nursing care. Nurs Health Sci. 2015;17(3):354–61.
112. Taguchi T, Yano M, Kido Y. Influence of bright light therapy on postoperative patients: a pilot study. Intensive Crit Care Nurs. 2007;23(5):289–97.
113. Simons KS, et al. Dynamic light application therapy to reduce the incidence and duration of delirium in intensive-care patients: a randomised controlled trial. Lancet Respir Med. 2016;4(3):194–202.
114. Bannon L, et al. The effectiveness of non-pharmacological interventions in reducing the incidence and duration of delirium in critically ill patients: a systematic review and meta-analysis. Intensive Care Med. 2019;45(1):1–12.
115. Davidson JE, et al. Guidelines for family-centered care in the neonatal, pediatric, and adult ICU. Crit Care Med. 2017;45(1):103–28.
116. Knutsson S, Golsäter M, Enskär K. The meaning of being a visiting child of a seriously ill parent receiving care at the ICU. Int J Qual Stud Health Well Being. 2021;16(1):1999884.
117. Munro CL, et al. Delirium prevention in critically ill adults through an automated reorientation intervention—a pilot randomized controlled trial. Heart Lung. 2017;46(4):234–8.
118. Brandao Barreto B, et al. Exploring patients' perceptions on ICU diaries: a systematic review and qualitative data synthesis. Crit Care Med. 2021;49(7):E707–18.
119. Wilson ME, et al. Humanizing the intensive care unit. Crit Care. 2019;23(1):32.
120. Bohart S, et al. Perspectives and wishes for patient and family centred care as expressed by adult intensive care survivors and family-members: a qualitative interview study. Intensive Crit Care Nurs. 2023;75:103346.
121. Hosey MM, et al. Animal-assisted intervention in the ICU: a tool for humanization. Crit Care. 2018;22(1):22.
122. Chlan LL, et al. Effects of patient-directed music intervention on anxiety and sedative exposure in critically ill patients receiving mechanical ventilatory support: a randomized clinical trial. JAMA. 2013;309(22):1–10.
123. Hetland B, Lindquist R, Chlan LL. The influence of music during mechanical ventilation and weaning from mechanical ventilation: a review. Heart Lung. 2015;44(5):416–25.
124. Hansen IP, Langhorn L, Dreyer P. Effects of music during daytime rest in the intensive care unit: effect of music in the ICU. Nurs Crit Care. 2018;23(4):207–13.

Psychology: Person-Centred Care a Key to Successful Recovery

10

Julie Highfield, Matthew Beadman, and Dorothy Wade

10.1 Introduction: Patient Experience and Psychological Stressors in the ICU

A significant number of patients are admitted to adult, general critical care units across Europe, with an average of 208,000 annual admissions in the UK in 2019–2021 [1]. Although medical advances lead to an increasing number of people surviving their critical care admission, there is evidence many critical care patients develop both acute and long-term psychological difficulties [2]. Critical care or intensive care units (ICUs) are often described by patients as stressful places, where they may suffer pain, thirst, hunger, nausea, fatigue, discomfort and disorientation associated with critical illness, invasive medical procedures and monitoring, and side-effects of potent drugs [3]. As many critical care patients are likely to have multiple invasive procedures, there is a danger of some patients being re-traumatised repeatedly. Mechanical ventilation has been identified as a risk factor for psychological difficulties in some but not all studies [4] and a meta-ethnography of 38 qualitative studies highlighted how frightening this was, using illustrative patient quotes such as,

You know, if you need it, and it does a good job and it helps you, I suppose the misery is worth it. But I would offer this as a good torture for Guantanamo. [5]

J. Highfield
University Hospital Wales, Cardiff, Wales, UK
e-mail: Julie.Highfield@wales.nhs.uk

M. Beadman
Independent Practice, Guildford, Surrey, UK
e-mail: matthew@rethinkhealth-online.com

D. Wade (✉)
Royal Free London NHS Foundation Trust, London, UK
e-mail: dorothy.wade@nhs.net

© The Author(s), under exclusive license to Springer Nature Switzerland AG 2024
C. Boulanger, D. McWilliams (eds.), *Passport to Successful Outcomes for Patients Admitted to ICU*, https://doi.org/10.1007/978-3-031-53019-7_10

In one study, the Therapeutic Intervention Scoring System (TISS, a measure of increasing amount of critical care interventions delivered) was associated with increased risk of post-traumatic stress disorder (PTSD) [4].

Being attached to organ support machines, tubes, masks, lines, drips and other equipment in a busy and noisy ward often without access to daylight, windows or clocks, can lead to sensory overload but paradoxically also to sensory deprivation, circadian rhythm dysregulation and sleep deprivation. A large body of research attests that patients in ICUs often feel isolated, alienated and unable to communicate (due to the endotracheal tube or to surgery), but all too aware of other people's suffering or death in their vicinity [6]. It is perhaps no surprise that 45–80% of critical care patients experience acute stress in the form of panic, fear, anxiety, depressed mood, anger, irritability or frightening nightmares, hallucinations or delusions [2, 7, 8]. Hallucinations and delusions are reported to occur in the context of delirium, a syndrome consisting of cognitive deficits, attentional deficits, psychomotor disturbance, circadian rhythm disturbance and emotional dysregulation, which affects up to 80% of mechanically ventilated patients and up to 50% of non-ventilated patients (see Fig. 10.1) [9, 10]. For a diagnosis of delirium, there must be evidence that the cause is not another medical condition, substance intoxication, substance withdrawal or exposure to a toxin. The pathophysiology of delirium is still unclear, but

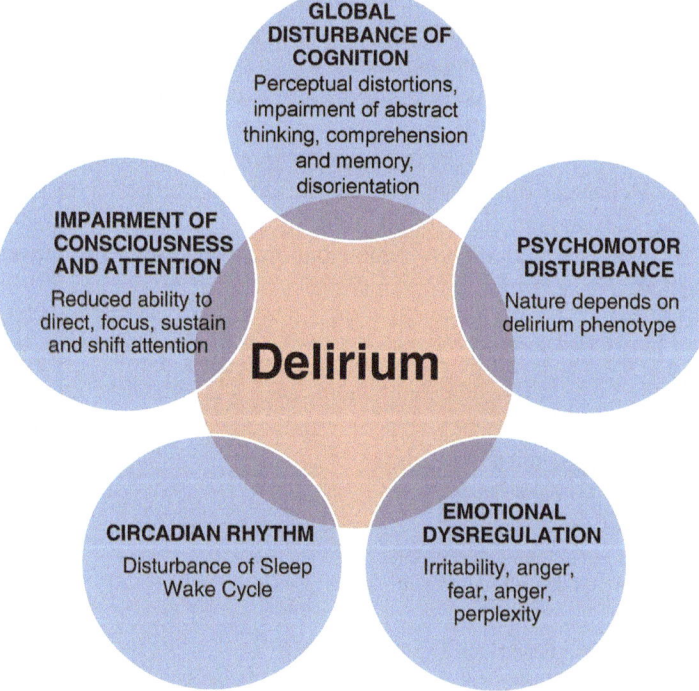

Fig. 10.1 Five core domains of delirium [9]

hypotheses include inflammation, physiological stress, and disruption to the processes of cerebral metabolism and neurotransmission [9]. More recently, these hypotheses have been drawn together by a more sophisticated theory that arises from the latest neuroscience of neural networks. Chemical imbalances caused by drugs, inflammation, infection or others may prevent the brain from switching smoothly between two key neural networks, the attention and default mode networks, giving rise to the variable range of symptoms of delirium, from inattention to memory problems to hallucinations and delusions [11].

Many patients receive a cocktail of psychoactive drugs in critical care units, including opioids to deal with pain, benzodiazepines to manage anxiety, hypnotics for sleep and sedatives/anaesthetics to tolerate mechanical ventilation. It is now recognised that iatrogenic coma and immobilisation are harmful to patients, leading to delirium, long-term cognitive impairment, ICU-acquired weakness, and psychological difficulties such as depression and PTSD. As a result, critical care units now aim to keep patients more lightly sedated and to stop sedation as soon as possible, but over-sedation of patients remains common [12].

10.2   Post-ICU Psychological Outcomes and Risk Factors

Studies indicate that as many as 50% of patients develop symptoms of anxiety, depression or post-traumatic stress disorder (see Table 10.1), in the months or years after leaving a critical care unit [4, 13]. Patients with post-ICU post-traumatic stress symptoms may experience flashbacks and intrusive memories of delusional/hallucinatory episodes from delirium as well as actual events within the ICU [8, 14]. Patients may also experience persistent cognitive changes with problems in functions such as attention, memory and executive function. Both psychological health difficulties and cognitive changes are important domains of post-intensive care syndrome (PICS, see Fig. 10.2), along with the third domain of physical issues [2].

A history of psychological difficulties, use of benzodiazepines and duration of sedation are risk factors (see Table 10.2) for adverse ICU psychological outcomes [15]. Both acute stress and memories of delirious experiences in the ICU have also been identified as potential risk factors. Acute ICU stress is associated with post-discharge anxiety, depression, PTSD, cognitive changes and increased alcohol use [4, 18] while memories of delirious experiences are associated with PTSD and

Table 10.1 Psychological and cognitive difficulties following critical illness

Psychological	Neurocognitive
Depression	Delirium
Anxiety disorders	Persistent cognitive impairment—commonly in executive function, memory, attention and word finding
Post-traumatic stress disorder	
Adjustment reactions	

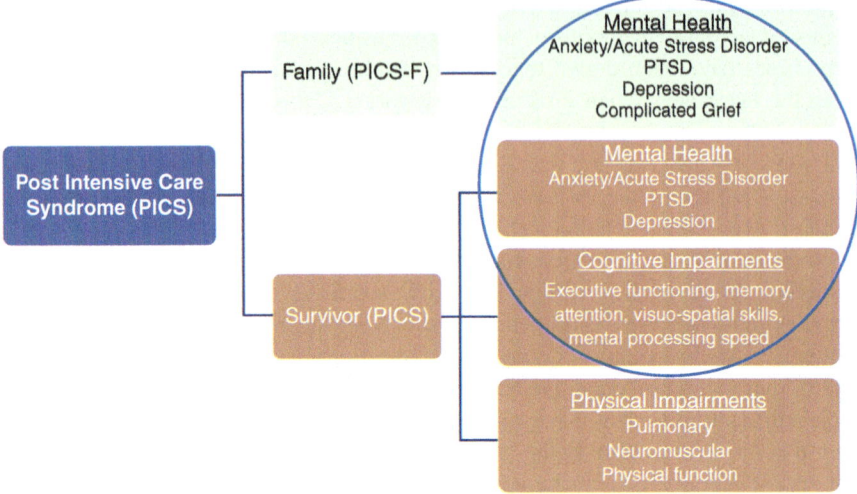

Fig. 10.2 Psychological domains of post-intensive care syndrome [13]

Table 10.2 Modifiable and static risk factors for psychological and cognitive difficulties following critical illness

Modifiable risk factors	Static risk factors
Acute stress in the ICU [4]	Pre-existing mental health problems [14]
Longer duration of sedation [4]	Type of illness: ARDS/sepsis [15]
Longer period of delirium [16, 17]	Younger age [17]
Use of inotropes or vasopressors [4]	Lower education level [15]
Use of benzodiazepines [4, 14]	Previous history of psychological health difficulties [15]
Mood in the ICU [4]	Female sex
Early intrusive memories of the ICU [14]	Lower socio-economic status [4]
Distressed behaviour and use of restraint [15]	

depression [8]. Therefore, delirious experiences and acute stress may be modifiable factors that could be reduced to prevent subsequent psychological difficulties.

The role of delirious experiences/memories in the development of post-ICU psychological difficulties is not yet clear, and delirium was not found to be associated with PTSD in a well-conducted cohort study of 567 patients [19]. However more recent studies have shown an association between ICU delirium and worse mental health outcomes including anxiety, depression and PTSD [20, 21]. ICU delirium is also a risk factor for cognitive difficulties, and a multi-centre, prospective cohort study of 821 ICU survivors identified several types of delirium (sedative-related, hypoxic, septic and unclassified delirium) that were associated with worse cognitive function at 12 months [16].

Screening tools are now available to detect both delirium and acute stress in Intensive Care patients. The CAM-ICU is the most commonly used tool to detect delirium in the ICU [10]. A screening tool to detect acute stress in ICU patients, the Intensive Care Psychological Assessment Tool (IPAT) has been developed and validated [22] and is now used in a number of UK and international critical care units.

10.3 Early Interventions Addressing Delirium/ Cognitive Changes in the ICU

Sedatives or antipsychotics are often prescribed in the Intensive Care Unit to address acute stress and delirium, but they have potentially harmful side-effects, both physical and psychological [12]. Environmental interventions to reduce triggers of fear and stress in the Intensive Care unit would seem to offer a preventative approach to both delirium and acute stress. Triggers include being unable to communicate, having thirst or hunger, being woken up by care activities at night, loud or alarming noise, unnatural light, crowding around the bedside, shapes and shadows at nighttime, missing one's family and many others [23].

In ICU, distressed behaviour is often managed by administering haloperidol, quetiapine or olanzapine. Yet, literature from geriatric medicine highlights that side effects of anti-psychotic medications are particularly problematic in elderly patients [24] and emphasises the need for staff to always look for a reason for the behaviour as the first step. Causative factors include patients who can't communicate normally becoming distressed because they have unmet needs such as pain, discomfort, hunger, thirst, frustration, boredom, lack of social contact, isolation, feeling frightened, disorientated or threatened or unable to find loved ones. To help, staff should aim to assess the root cause of the patients' distress and attempt to meet their needs—well before a patient's behaviour becomes so challenging that it is a threat to their own or others' safety. Other causes include environments that are either under- or over-stimulating (and ICUs can often, paradoxically, be both of these things). A third common cause is where patients perceive they are receiving inadequate staff attention or where staff behaviour may be perceived as not person-centred [24].

Humanistic person-centred care is key to all staff-patient communication but is even more important when dealing with distressed or delirious patients. Originally conceived by Carl Rogers [25], person-centred care promotes key values and attitudes such as warmth, genuineness, unconditional positive regard (acceptance), empathic understanding and non-judgmentalism. This approach is strongly promoted in the care of mental health patients with psychotic disorders such as schizophrenia. This field of healthcare has much to offer to the care of intensive care patients, particularly regarding therapeutic communication with people having unusual experiences such as hallucinations and delusions. For example, a large qualitative review [26] encapsulated evidence and advice from nurses who are expert in caring for this population. Patients are often reluctant to share unusual experiences because of not wanting to cause a fuss, being worried that people will

Table 10.3 Communication tips for critical care staff working with patients with delirium and distress [23, 27]

Setting the scene
Be person-centred, i.e. warm, genuine, accepting, understanding, non-judgemental
Build rapport—be open, honest and listening to gain trust
Acknowledge that ICU is distressing, and that discussing worries is difficult
Discuss emotions with sensitivity
Aim to assess root causes of distressed behaviour, and address unmet needs, e.g. pain, thirst, loneliness
What to do
Have open, visible body language and give hallucinating patients lots of personal space
Use caring tone of voice and manner when discussing worries and fears
Use slow speech, simple vocabulary and short sentences
If a verbal patient is speaking rapidly, then slow down the pace of conversation
Talk to patients with hallucinations and delusions as rational people with unusual experiences
If challenged by patients to confirm a delusion, then say it seems unlikely to you, but you are open to learning otherwise
Acknowledge the stress that unusual experiences can cause for patients,and emphasise that your priority is helping them feel calm and safe
What not to do
Make gestures that look like ordering/criticising—pointing, arm-folding or finger-wagging
Allow your voice to sound frustrated or irritable
Laugh at hallucinations and delusions
Contradict, dismiss or minimise delusions
Encourage paranoia
Use phrases that sound patronising or sarcastic

think they are 'mad' and delusional fears such as '*the hospital is a prison camp*' and hopelessness or depression. Openness, honesty and listening are the tools needed to build rapport and persuade patients to open up. Attention should be paid to paraverbal, nonverbal as well as verbal aspects of communication. Table 10.3 includes the best tips for communicating with distressed and delirious people. The focus is on staff not behaving in a way that is unintentionally frightening; not arguing with patient's delusions, while not encouraging paranoia; stressing that staff are there to help them feel comfortable and safe. Further research needs to be carried out to evaluate these types of approach in critical care.

Multi-modal interventions to reduce delirium in the ICU currently offer the greatest potential for protecting patients from cognitive (and potentially mental health) difficulties post-discharge. The ABCDEF bundle [28] provides evidence-based strategies to combat the adverse effects of critical illness related to neurological dysfunction, which includes (1) assess, prevent and manage pain; (2) both spontaneous awakening trials and spontaneous breathing trials; (3) choice of analgesia and sedation; (4) delirium: assess, manage and treat; (5) early mobility and exercise and (6) family engagement and empowerment.

However the ABCDEF bundle does not fully address the emotional/psychological component of delirium—although it is one of five key domains in Maldonado's 2017 model (Fig. 10.1) [9]. In fact, psychological management of delirium has long been advocated [29]. This would include psychology-led consultations to reduce delirium incidence post-surgery, coordination of environmental, emotional, behavioural and cognitive interventions for delirium, and gentle reality testing of hallucinations and delusions for patients who have readiness for that intervention.

Interestingly, the new SIGN (Scottish Intercollegiate Guidelines Network) delirium guidelines [30] include psychological interventions such as (a) assess causes of and treat agitation and/or distress, using non-pharmacological means only if possible and (b) promote cognitive engagement and other rehabilitation strategies, within

Table 10.4 Non-pharmacological delirium risk reduction and treatment (Scottish Intercollegiate Guidelines Network) [30] (Psycho-social elements highlighted in bold)

Risk reduction
The following components should be considered as part of a package of care for patients at risk of developing delirium:
• **Orientation and ensuring patients have their glasses and hearing aids**
• **Promoting sleep hygiene (including use of ear plugs)**
• Early mobilisation
• Pain control
• Prevention, early identification and treatment of post-operative complications
• Maintaining optimal hydration and nutrition
• Regulation of bladder and bowel function
• Provision of supplementary oxygen, if appropriate
• **Ward moves should be avoided wherever possible for patients at risk of delirium**
• **Prior to surgery, patients and carers should be advised of the risk of developing delirium, to alleviate distress and help with management if it does occur**
• **Where possible, assistance should be sought from a patients' relatives and carers to deliver care to reduce the risk of delirium developing**
• Anaesthetic management: depth of anaesthesia should be monitored in all patients aged over 60 years under general anaesthesia for surgery expected to last for more than 1 h, with the aim of avoiding excessively deep anaesthesia
Treatment
Healthcare professionals should follow established pathways of good care to manage patients with delirium:
• First consider acute, life-threatening causes of delirium including low oxygen level, low blood pressure, low glucose level and drug intoxication or withdrawal
• Systematically identify and treat potential causes (medications, acute illness, etc.) noting that multiple causes are common
• Optimise physiology, management of concurrent conditions, **environment (reduce noise), medications and natural sleep to promote brain recovery**
• **Specifically detect/assess causes of, and treat agitation and/or distress using non-pharmacological means only, if possible**
• **Communicate the diagnosis to patients and carers, encourage involvement of carers and provide ongoing engagement and support**
• Aim to prevent complications of delirium such as immobility, falls, pressure sores, dehydration, malnourishment and isolation
• Monitor for recovery and consider specialist referral if not recovering
• **Consider follow-up**
• **Promote cognitive engagement, mobilisation and other rehabilitation strategies**

their non-pharmacological bundles for delirium risk reduction and treatment (see Table 10.4) and of course, the emphasis should be on risk reduction, as there is still no treatment for ICU delirium whose effectiveness has been established [31, 32].

10.4 Assessment and Interventions for Acute Stress in the ICU

Given the severity of the interacting physical, psychological and social stressors that patients commonly experience upon waking in the ICU, it is important to begin screening, assessing and addressing risk factors for psychological difficulties and sub-optimal rehabilitation outcomes from an early stage. A National Institute for

Table 10.5 Author recommendations for applied psychology for NICE (QS158) Statements 1–4

Quality statement (QS)	Recommendations for applied psychology
QS1: Adults in critical care at risk of morbidity have their rehabilitation goals agreed within 4 days of admission to critical care or before discharge from critical care, whichever is earlier[a] QS2. Adults at risk of morbidity have a formal handover of their care including their agreed individualised structured rehabilitation programme, when they transfer from critical care to a general ward[a]	– Organising the screening of psychological distress using the Intensive Care Psychological Assessment Tool (IPAT) [22] – For patients at risk of morbidity, perform a comprehensive assessment to identify current concerns and needs. – Provision of non-pharmacological interventions for delirium – Consider opening a patient diary – Application of principles of Psychological First Aid to increase feelings of safeness – Psychoeducation about the cause and meaning of hallucinations and delusions – Consider treating acute stress/lack of engagement within a CBT model
QS3: Adults who were in critical care and at risk of morbidity are given information based on their rehabilitation goals before they are discharged from hospital	– Provision of accessible information about a patient's illness, what happened to them and emotional reactions (verbally, and in written form, to take home) – Cognitive Behavioural approaches to address acute stress/lack of engagement
QS4: Adults who stayed in critical care for more than 4 days and were at risk of morbidity have a review 2–3 months after discharge from critical care	– Participation in ICU follow-up clinics – Provision of outpatient evidence-based psychological therapies and cognitive assessment/rehabilitation when required – Signposting to peer support, stress management, mindfulness or other appropriate groups

[a] The timing of delivery of the recommendations for applied psychology under Quality Standard 1 and 2 will depend on individual cases

Health and Care Excellence (NICE) guideline [33] has recommended that critical care patients suffering acute stress should be identified and offered psychological support as part of their structured rehabilitation plan. A 2017 NICE quality standard [34] was implemented to strengthen these requirements (see Table 10.5 for our recommendations for psychology input for each of the four quality statements). However, due to a lack of evidence about what helps, efforts to alleviate critical care patients' stressful experiences are variable in practice.

The Faculty of Intensive Care Medicine [UK] General Provision of Intensive Care Services GPICS-2 [35] recommends all critical care units should have practitioner psychologists to coordinate psychological assessments and interventions, and a growing number of these expert staff have been employed. As previously mentioned, the Intensive Care Psychological Assessment Tool (IPAT) [22] has been validated as a screening measure of early acute stress on the ICU and contains ten items assessing quality of sleep, communication, anxiety, low mood, experience of hallucinations, delusions and early traumatic memories. Scores above seven (range 0–20) indicate a need for further psychological assessment and/or interventions.

A systematic review [36] of the efficacy of early interventions to prevent the onset of PTSD in survivors of life-threatening medical events included 21 studies ($n = 4486$) and considered a range of psychological, pharmacological and behavioural interventions. Nine of these studies assessed interventions in ICU patients including CBT, mindfulness training, the provision of earplugs and eye masks, ICU diaries, the introduction of a rehabilitation workbook, comparing depths of sedation and intensifying rehabilitation resources. The review offers preliminary but not strong evidence that some psychological and pharmacological interventions may prevent the onset of PTSD. There was minimal evidence that early interventions can be harmful.

Similarly, a systematic review of non-pharmacological interventions to reduce acute stress in the ICU [37] identified 23 studies including 15 RCTs, of which 12 found the intervention to be beneficial. However, the quality of evidence was deemed to be weak to moderate. Promising interventions included music and nature-sounds therapy for ventilated patients, which reduced both psychological and physiological stress, and mind-body therapies such as acupressure. Some psychological interventions were found to be effective. In particular, an Italian study of 209 trauma patients [38] found that introducing a clinical psychology service to the ICU significantly reduced PTSD and the use of psychiatric medication at 6 months. It was reported that each patient received on average five or six clinical psychology interventions including stress management techniques such as cognitive restructuring and coping strategies for families and patients. However, the pre- and post-historical control study design was weak, and it is not possible to elucidate which interventions were carried out most frequently or were most helpful.

Within the broader psychological trauma literature, trauma-focused Cognitive-Behavioural Therapy (CBT) is the frontline treatment for Acute Stress Disorder, defined as experiencing a traumatic event and having dissociative, re-experiencing, avoidance and arousal symptoms, which cause significant distress or impairment and last for a minimum of 2 days and maximum of 4 weeks [39]. While trauma-focused CBT is explicitly recommended by NICE (NG116) [40] as a preventative treatment for PTSD, necessary preconditions such as the absence of perceived threat or danger, intact cognition and an appropriate environment may preclude the majority of ICU patients from receiving this.

Although not explicitly written about in a critical care context, trauma literature suggests that principles from Psychological First Aid (PFA) [41] can be drawn upon to help foster feelings of safeness. PFA is an internationally applied evidence-informed approach to helping people affected by a traumatic incident, which is designed to reduce acute distress and foster adaptive coping. PFA provides key actions that healthcare providers can apply to help people feel safer and to facilitate adaptive coping, including reassurance through normalising, helping people reunite with loved ones and enabling voluntary sharing of experiences.

Elements of PFA and CBT were combined in an intervention aiming to reduce acute stress and other risk factors of PTSD that were evaluated in the POPPI trial [42], a multi-centre, parallel-group, cluster-randomised clinical trial involving 1453 patients. Participants screened as having acute stress in units randomised to the intervention, received a three-session nurse-led psychological intervention based on elements of CBT for psychosis [43], which aimed to reduce stress, including distress related to hallucinations and delusions. Selected nurses received 3 days of training to deliver the three-session intervention. In intervention units, online training was also provided to all staff to make changes to the ICU environment to promote therapeutic value, and to improve communication between staff and distressed patients. Primary outcome was self-reported PTSD severity at 6 months and secondary outcomes included number of days alive and free of sedation, anxiety, depression and quality of life. However, no significant differences in these outcomes were found between the intervention and control groups. The lack of effectiveness of the POPPI intervention may be due to timing too early, which did not enable full use of CBT protocols used elsewhere, dosage, complexity and whether such interventions are better delivered by practitioner psychologists [44].

Roles for psychologists in ICU have been explored, e.g. Bennun [45] suggested key aims for a clinical psychologist working in ICU to be reducing social isolation, establishing a day-night cycle, engaging in communication with the patient, involving family, and using cognitive approaches to treating anxiety, hallucinations and delusions. Other interesting approaches include the use of positive suggestions for ventilated, sedated patients [46] and existentialist psychotherapy sessions to explore the meaning of hallucinations and delusions [47]. Sideris [47] suggests that sometimes psychologists just being present and sitting in silence with a non-verbal patient, or showing that they care about the 'awfulness' of a patient's experience, can be powerful therapeutic tools. Cohen et al. [48] report on a case series of ventilator dependent patients successfully weaned with cognitive behavioural therapy.

Few psychological intervention studies have focused on reducing depression as a primary outcome. One study [17] found higher rates of depression (33% at 12 months) than PTSD (7%), with somatic symptoms of depression significantly more commonly reported than cognitive symptoms. This finding has important implications for assessment since anti-depressants tend to be less helpful for somatic symptoms of depression. Physical rehabilitation and behavioural activation may offer scope for improvement, consistent with recommendations (NICE CG90) [49]. Behavioural activation implemented by occupational therapists to address depressive symptoms and physical function after acute respiratory failure is currently being evaluated by Dr. Ann Parker in the USA (ClinicalTrials.gov identifier NCT03431493).

Physical exercise also features in combination with cognitive rehabilitation in intra-ICU interventions developed to improve cognitive outcomes of ICU. The Activity and Cognitive Therapy in the ICU trial [50] demonstrated the feasibility of providing both cognitive and physical rehabilitation for mechanically ventilated patients during their ICU admission. The Measuring Outcomes of Activity in Intensive Care (MOSAIC) study (ClinicalTrials.gov identifier NCT03115840) aims to assess the effects of activity during an ICU admission on physical and cognitive functioning following discharge.

Intra-ICU strategies should also consider the psychological needs of family members and friends. Lee et al. [51] assessed the impact of protocol-driven family support interventions on length of stay in intensive care through a systematic review and meta-analysis. Seven randomised and controlled trials were included ($n = 3477$). The family support interventions primarily aimed to enhance communication between family members and medical teams and were effective in reducing ICU length of stay in critically ill patients without impacting mortality. The review suggests that providing leaflets and educational materials is likely to be ineffective unless combined with offering family members time to ask questions and emphasises the importance of empathetic and trusting relationships. Rosa et al. [52] report the ICU visits randomised clinical trial, which investigated whether a flexible visitation policy in the ICU supported by family education reduces the incidence of delirium. Flexible visitation did not significantly reduce the incidence of delirium but was associated with reduced psychological distress in family members as a secondary outcome.

10.5 Leaving the ICU

To help patients make sense of what has happened to them during an ICU admission, critical care teams routinely provide patients and their families with healthcare information. However, a range of factors pose a barrier to the retention of information including pain, sleep deprivation, the effects of medication, anxiety and confusion. Bench et al. [53] evaluated the feasibility and effectiveness of a written information ICU discharge pack, which aimed to improve early rehabilitation from critical illness. Although underpowered with 158 participants, this study provides preliminary data that written discharge information based on Leventhal's self-regulation theory is feasible and may help to optimise rehabilitation [53].

The authors were unable to find studies of psychological interventions for patients on other hospital wards following critical care discharge (although many stress support sessions were delivered on other wards in the POPPI study). However, further research would be beneficial, as the post-ICU hospitalisation period may provide patients with the space, time and privacy needed to reflect on and process ICU experiences.

10.6   Going Home

When a patient leaves the ward to go home, they continue their journey of recovery, but with closer access to their own resources and support systems of family, friends and home. In our experience, on the return home patients will need to negotiate their own and others' expectations about recovery. Patient stories include those of frustration and concern at not returning to everyday life as quickly as they might expect, as well as managing ongoing limits in their functioning, such as being slowed down cognitively and physically. At some point the patients are likely to reach their maximum level of functioning, which may be a lower baseline than pre-admission. As patients make sense of the difference between their pre-hospital baseline and their new baseline, they are likely to go through a period of psychological adjustment. For many, as we have seen, there are a range of ongoing psychological difficulties including anxiety, depression, post-traumatic stress disorder, cognitive problems such as poor memory, and family and relationship issues, collectively known as PICS (Fig. 10.2). In a bid to tackle PICS, there is a growing literature on post-ICU interventions, including follow-up clinics, peer support groups, group psychological interventions and individual psychological interventions.

10.7   Follow-Up Clinics

With growing evidence of problems post-discharge home, there are supporting guidelines on the expected response of the ICU. NICE Guidance CG83 [33] recommends a multi-disciplinary follow-up clinic for patients post-ICU, a recommendation further supported in the GPICS 2 [35], which supports the provision of trained practitioner psychologists to provide psychological interventions to patients following discharge home. However, despite this, there is very limited evidence to demonstrate the effectiveness of follow-up clinics. For example, Cuthbertson et al. [54] undertook a non-blinded multi-centre randomised controlled trial of nurse-led ICU follow-up clinics across three hospitals recruiting 286 patients (192 at 1 year follow-up), with no difference at 12 months in health-related quality of life. These clinics were found to be significantly more costly than standard care and therefore not considered to be cost-effective. A recent systematic review of follow-up clinics suggests research is thus far inconclusive, although the authors note the sparsity of research and the variation in delivery of clinics [55].

From experience, however, we might argue that single-session follow-up clinics allow for the screening of post-intensive care syndrome and signposting on to necessary interventions; therefore, such clinics are unlikely to provide an effective intervention in and of themselves. Some suggest that this is a service that could be better provided by GPs, especially if communication between intensive care units and GPs was improved [56]. However patient-reported experience indicates perceived benefits from attending a follow-up clinic; for example, it is a chance for them to ask questions about their stay and make sense of what happened to them, and it can allow them to reduce their anxieties regarding ongoing risk of recurrence and understand unusual symptoms.

In the InS:PIRE study, McPeake et al. [57] followed up 49 selected patients from one ICU in Scotland, offering a five-week peer-supported rehabilitation programme. This multidisciplinary programme included pharmacy, physiotherapy, nursing, medical and psychology input. Forty patients completed follow-up surveys at 12 months with a positive improvement in quality of life for those patients who took part in the intervention compared to historical controls. Self-efficacy improved over the duration of the five-week programme and was sustained at one year post-intervention. Eighty-eight percent returned to employment or volunteering compared to 46% in the control group [57].

10.8   Return of Patient Diaries

One function of the follow-up clinic can be to return an ICU Diary, an initiative where staff and relatives complete a layman's account during the intensive care stay that is then returned to the patient after they have been discharged; the original rationale was to fill a memory gap of the ICU admission, something that many patients struggle to recall, as a preventative intervention for post-traumatic stress [58]. Many units use this initiative, and a European group has developed bringing together all of the literature (http://www.icu-diary.org). Garrouste-Orgeas et al. [59] designed the ICU-Diary Study as a multi-centre, randomised, parallel and controlled study to assess the impact of the ICU diary on the psychological wellbeing of both patients and families 3 months post-ICU discharge in 367 patients. There was no difference between the control and intervention groups; therefore the findings do not support the use of an ICU diary as preventative of PTSD. However, there seems to be a diverse range of opinions from ICU patients and their families about the utility of the ICU diary, suggesting a potential range of mechanisms to aid recovery, and that some patients benefit while others do not; perhaps, the focus should be wider than only evaluating their effectiveness in the prevention of PTSD [60].

10.9   Peer Support Groups

Another way of providing follow-up to patients is via peer support groups, although there is limited published evidence for the effectiveness of these groups. The UK charity ICU Steps supports a five-step methodology to develop post-ICU support groups for patients. An international review of support groups found six models of peer support (community-based, psychologist-led outpatient, models within ICU follow-up clinics, groups within the ICU, peer mentorships and online). These groups experience common barriers to sustainability, including funding, risk management, personnel and recruitment [61]. It has been suggested that perhaps patients do not see themselves as survivors of ICU, but as survivors of their specific accident or illness, and as such these groups are not offering the peer support required [62].

Such programmes of ICU follow-up and peer support are considered to also have benefit to the clinicians providing ICU care. In a qualitative study of clinician's views of post-ICU follow-up and peer support, the reciprocal nature of such programmes was identified, such as a feedback loop for quality improvement, increasing awareness in clinicians and improving the meaningfulness of ICU work [63].

10.10 Psychological Interventions

A small number of researchers have trialled post-ICU specific psychological interventions with mixed results. Jensen et al. [64] describe a nurse-led post-hospital recovery program where patients were given a journal of their ICU stay and three follow-up consultations (the RAPIT study a pragmatic, non-blinded, multicentre, parallel-group RCT across ten Danish ICUs). There was no difference in health-related quality of life, depression, PTSD or utilisation of services, although there was some reduction in anxiety in the intervention group.

A 3-month mindfulness programme was found to be feasible and acceptable to post-ICU patients whether delivered by phone (with a therapist) or by a mobile telephone App [65]. The same team developed a 6-week psychologist-delivered telephone based coping skills training (CST) programme based on cognitive behavioural therapy principles [66]. The CST included the following six stages: (1) introduction and relaxation exercise, (2) progressive muscle relaxation, (3) pleasant activities and activity–rest cycle, (4) communication, (5) cognitive restructuring and pleasant imagery and (6) review and planning for sustainability. The CST did not improve psychological distress symptoms compared with an education programme, but did improve symptoms of distress at 6 months among patients with high baseline distress, whereas the education program improved distress at 3 months among those ventilated for more than 7 days.

One of the most common psychological concerns following ICU discharge is the experience of post-traumatic stress disorder (PTSD). NICE guidance for the treatment and management of PTSD indicates the effectiveness of psychological therapies [40]. However, some patients post-ICU may struggle to access services for PTSD due to stringent diagnostic criteria. Brewin [67] recently commented that in the American Psychiatric Association's Diagnostic and Statistical Manual of Mental Disorders (DSM-5), a diagnosis of PTSD requires an objectively traumatic event that involves exposure to death or threat of death or serious injury, and therefore potentially neglects groups of patients who experience a triggering event that is subjectively traumatic. The experience of delirium and associated hallucinations and delusions of threat and harm in ICU present no objective threat, but the lived experience of patients is very real, and some continue to consider the memory to be real despite knowing that it did not happen to them.

One recommended psychological therapy is Eye Movement Desensitisation and Reprocessing (EMDR), an approach that facilitates the accessing and processing of traumatic or adverse memories through asking the person to attend to this material while simultaneously focusing on a therapist-directed external stimulus such as lateral eye movements. Hulme [68] undertook a small pilot trial of EMDR with ten patients post-ICU, with positive reductions in PTSD and depressive symptoms in an average of five sessions, suggesting potential for further exploration for post-ICU related PTSD. Bates and colleagues undertook a feasibility trial for the Recent Traumatic Event Protocol for EMDR delivered online for patients admitted for COVID-19. In the post-ICU period, they found PTSD symptom reduction in the treatment group, albeit in a very small sample (11 in intervention group vs. 12 controls), indicating that EMDR is feasible and acceptable to patients post-ICU although clearly more work is needed [69]. Other NICE-recommended approaches to PTSD include types of trauma-focused Cognitive-Behavioural Therapy such as cognitive processing, narrative therapy, cognitive therapy for PTSD and prolonged exposure [40]. There are no other published studies of trauma-focused psychological therapies specific to the post-ICU population. The authors are aware of ongoing studies that are not yet published (e.g. the PICTURE trial in Germany of GP-delivered, psychologist supervised 3-session Narrative Therapy for PTSD post-ICU (ISRCTN registry 97280643) and a Cambridge, UK case-control study of an intervention based on CBT and narrative exposure therapy (NET) for PTSD).

It is notable that many of the interventions described are new or innovative programmes of intervention, and are often nurse-led. Little has been published about individual psychological therapies offered to patients post-ICU. It may be that many ICU survivors present to primary and secondary mental health services and despite the lack of research evidence to support post-ICU specific interventions, there is plenty of evidence to suggest the efficacy of psychological therapies. NICE guidance suggests the efficacy of psychological therapies for depression [49] and various sub-types of anxiety disorder [70], including low intensity psychological therapies such as computerised CBT, guided self-help and group-based CBT, and high intensity psychological therapies such as CBT, Interpersonal Therapy, behavioural couples therapy, and short-term psychodynamic psychotherapy. More research is required to prove the efficacy of these therapies when applied specifically to target symptoms of PICS.

10.11   Cognitive Interventions

A single, small, randomised controlled study of 21 patients, showed that a post-ICU cognitive, physical and functional individual rehabilitation intervention had an effect in improving cognitive performance [71]. The cognitive component provided six 1–1 contacts of cognitive rehabilitation exercises based on a Goal Management Protocol which targets patient executive functioning. Patients are encouraged to increase goal-directed behaviour while learning to be reflective ('stop and think') about consequences to decisions and divide tasks into manageable units. A limited proof-of-concept study of 24 patients used 18 computerised brain-training exercises to aid cognitive rehabilitation and showed an improvement in attention, processing speed, memory and executive function [72]. Larger cognitive intervention studies are needed and the IMPROVE study [73]—a four-arm randomised clinical trial, is underway to evaluate the efficacy of physical exercise and cognitive training on cognitive function among patients aged 50 years and older who experienced delirium during an ICU admission.

10.12 The Psychological Impact and Outcomes of ICU During and Post-COVID 19 in the UK

During the first two waves of mass hospitalisations due to the COVID-19 pandemic in 2020 and 2021, pre-vaccinations, the psychological impact of an admission to ICU appeared to be more severe than usual. Patients and families were separated, causing anxiety and isolation. Medical and psychological care from staff were affected by the large surges of patients into ICU, causing overcrowding and staff stress; and the need for staff to wear personal protective equipment covering bodies and faces, limiting communication. Excellent person-centred care and clinical communication were replaced by keeping patients more deeply sedated for longer periods.

Longer-term effects are mixed. Studies of long-term psychological impact on ICU patients with COVID-19 suggest similar rates of distress or neuro-psychiatric outcomes as in pre-COVID and non-COVID ICU patients [74]. On the positive side, media coverage of ICUs during COVID-19 highlighted issues such as ICU delirium and Post Intensive Care syndrome. This led to more funding in the UK for ICU psychology, and increased interest in multi-disciplinary rehabilitation and follow-up services. However, some of this funding proved to be temporary, and has not been translated into permanent psychology posts in the post-pandemic era. Similarly, the post-COVID follow-up clinics that were rapidly set up during the pandemic did not always lead to permanent ICU follow-up service funding.

Healthcare staff working during the pandemic experienced significant stress and burnout. For example, a sample of ICU staff reporting midway through the first wave of the pandemic indicated two fifths reported symptoms consistent with probable mental health diagnoses, including PTSD, anxiety and depression [75] which is an increase from pre-pandemic levels of approximately 13% [76]. This diagnostic approach has since come under scrutiny [77], but it is clear that staff turnover has been high in ICU since the pandemic [78]. In addition to the current impact on ICU staff, this level of distress also suggests workforce retention could be badly affected in the long term and impact patient care in ICU.

There remains a need to re-build, and build upon, excellent research and clinical experience in delivering person-centred care within a rehabilitation context, in ICUs of the future.

10.13   Conclusion

A wealth of research has documented that patients find ICU admissions highly stressful and that subsequently many survivors experience symptoms indicative of depression, anxiety, posttraumatic stress disorder and cognitive impairment. Work is underway to identify and modify risk factors for psychological and mental health difficulties, including sedation practices, delirious experiences and acute stress in the ICU. NICE now advocates psychological assessment and interventions for critically ill patients in and after their ICU admission, and the UK's Intensive Care Society supports the provision of senior practitioner psychologists in ICUs to oversee acute and follow-up psychological services, with a growing number of these expert staff now in place in UK ICUs. While high-quality evidence from randomised trials and systematic reviews is still lacking to support the precise form and mode of delivery of psychological support or therapy most beneficial for critically ill patients, promising interventions are being developed for each stage of the critical care patient's pathway (see Table 10.6). Interventions in the acute setting could include elements such as music therapy, complementary therapies, multi-disciplinary working to promote optimal rehabilitation, family psychoeducation programmes and evidence-based psychological approaches for delirium, and symptoms of acute stress. CBT treatments for trauma, anxiety and depression can be provided by specialist practitioner psychologists based in ICU follow-up services, who are

Table 10.6 Promising psychological interventions requiring further development and research

In the ICU
Cognitive-behavioural therapy (CBT) for ventilated patients [48]
Combined cognitive rehabilitation (goal management training) and physical therapy [50] for ventilated patients
Psychologist-led management of delirium and distressed behaviour [25–30]
Music therapy and complementary therapies to reduce acute stress in the ICU [37]
Psychologist-led relational approaches. Being present, acknowledging distress, exploring meaning and reducing isolation [45–48]
Use of clinical psychologists in the ICU to tackle distress and early trauma symptoms [38]
Nurse-led psychological support in the ICU [44]
Protocol-driven family support in the ICU [51]
OT-led behavioural activation to address symptoms of depression and physical function
Patient-friendly written information ICU discharge pack to improve early rehabilitation [53]
Post-ICU
Post-ICU mindfulness programme via telephone or mobile phone app [65]
Telephone based coping skills training (CST) programme delivered by clinical psychologist [66]
Intensive care patient diaries [60]
Eye movement desensitisation and reprocessing therapy for post-ICU patients with PTSD [68]
GP-led, psychologist-supervised narrative therapy for post-ICU PTSD (ongoing trial, unpublished)
Psychologist-led intervention for PTSD combining CBT and NET (unpublished)
5-week MDT rehabilitation programme [57]

familiar with the ICU context and embedded within multidisciplinary teams. Peer support, stress management or emotional regulation groups may also be run as adjunct services. Cognitive interventions for intensive care patients are starting to be developed but are still in their infancy. There is every hope that holistic person-centred care will increasingly become the norm in critical care services.

Key Take Home Messages
- ICU admission is often psychologically distressing.
- Delirium is a common factor in ICU-related distress.
- Distress within ICU predicts poor psychological outcome post-hospital discharge.
- Initial evidence supports the role of practitioner psychologists in mitigating ICU distress and managing post-ICU psychological sequelae.
- Further high-quality research is urgently needed in this area.

References

1. Intensive Care National Audit and Research Centre. The case mix programme summary statistics 2019/21. 2022. https://onlinereports.icnarc.org/Home. Accessed 2 Aug 2023.
2. Wade DM. Doctoral thesis: prevalence and predictors of psychological morbidity and quality of life after discharge from intensive care. London: University College; 2010.
3. Puntillo KA, Arai S, Cohen NH, Gropper MA, Neuhaus J, Paul SM, et al. Symptoms experienced by intensive care unit patients at high risk of dying. Crit Care Med. 2010;38(11):2155–60.
4. Wade DM, Howell DC, Weinman JA, Hardy RJ, Mythen MG, Brewin CR, et al. Investigating risk factors for psychological morbidity three months after intensive care: a prospective cohort study. Crit Care. 2012;16(5):R192.
5. Carruthers H, Gomershall T, Astin F. The work undertaken by mechanically ventilated patients in intensive care: a qualitative meta-ethnography of survivors' experiences. Int J Nurs Stud. 2018;86:60–73.
6. Alonso-Ovies A, Heras La Calle G. ICU: a branch of hell? Intensive Care Med. 2016;42(4):591–2.
7. Nelson JE. The symptom burden of chronic critical illness. Crit Care Med. 2004;32(7):1527–34.
8. Jones C, Backman C, Capuzzo M, Flaatten H, Rylander C, Griffiths RD. Precipitants of post-traumatic stress disorder following intensive care: a hypothesis generating study of diversity in care. Intensive Care Med. 2007;33(6):978–85.
9. Maldonado JR. Acute brain failure: pathophysiology, diagnosis, management, and sequelae of delirium. Crit Care Clin. 2017;33(3):461–519.
10. Ely EW, Inouye SK, Bernard GR, Gordon S, Francis J, May L. Delirium in mechanically ventilated patients: validity and reliability of the confusion assessment method for the intensive care unit (CAM-ICU). JAMA. 2001;286(21):2703–10.
11. Young JWS. The network model of delirium. Med Hypotheses. 2017;104:80–5.
12. Jackson JC, Santoro MJ, Ely TM, Boehm L, Keihl AL, Anderson LS, et al. Improving patient care through the prism of psychology: application of Maslow's hierarchy to sedation, delirium and early mobility in the ICU. J Crit Care. 2014;29(3):438–44.
13. Needham DM, Davidson J, Cohen H, Hopkins RO, Weinart C, Wunsch H, et al. Improving long-term outcomes after discharge from intensive care unit: report from a stakeholders' conference. Crit Care Med. 2012;40(2):502–9.
14. Wade DM, Brewin CR, Howell DC, White E, Mythen MG, Weinmart JA. Intrusive memories of hallucinations and delusions in traumatised intensive care patients: an interview study. Br J Health Psychol. 2015;20(3):613–31.

15. Davydow DS, Gifford JM, Desai SV, et al. Post-traumatic stress disorder in general intensive care survivors: a systematic review. Gen Hosp Psychiatry. 2008;30(5):421–34.
16. Pandharipande PP, Girard TD, Jackson JC, Morandi A, Thompson JL, Pun BT, et al. Long-term cognitive impairment after critical illness. N Engl J Med. 2013;369(14):1306–16.
17. Jackson JC, Pandharipande PP, Girard TD, Brummel NE, Thompson JL, Hughes CG. Depression, post-traumatic stress disorder, and functional disability in survivors of critical illness in the BRAIN-ICU study: a longitudinal cohort study. Lancet Respir Med. 2014;2(5):269–379.
18. Davydow DS, Zatzick D, Hough CL, Kanton WJ. In-hospital acute stress symptoms are associated with impairment in cognition 1 year after intensive care unit admission. Ann Am Thorac Soc. 2013;10(5):450–7.
19. Wolters AE, Peelen LA, Welling MC, Kok L, de Lange DW, Cremer OL, et al. Long term mental health problems after delirium in the Intensive Care Unit. Crit Care Med. 2016;44(10):1808–13.
20. Bulic D, Bennett M, Georgousopoulou EN, Shehabi Y, Pham T, Looi JCL, van Haren FMP. Cognitive and psychosocial outcomes of mechanically ventilated intensive care patients with and without delirium. Ann Intensive Care. 2020;10(1):104.
21. van der Heijden EFM, Kooken RWJ, Zegers M, Koen SS, van den Boogaard M. Differences in long-term outcomes between ICU patients with persistent delirium, non-persistent delirium and no delirium: a longitudinal cohort study. J Crit Care. 2023;76:2023.
22. Wade DM, Hankins M, Smyth DA, Rhone EE, Mythen MG, Howell DC, et al. Detecting acute distress and risk of future psychological morbidity in critically ill patients: validation of the intensive care psychological assessment tool. Crit Care. 2014;18(5):519.
23. Wade D, Als N, Bell V, Brewin C, D'Antoni D, Harrison DA, et al. Providing psychological support to people in critical care: development and feasibility study of a nurse-led intervention to prevent acute stress and long-term morbidity. BMJ Open. 2018;8(7):e021083.
24. Masand PS. Side effects of antipsychotics in the elderly. J Clin Psychiatry. 2000;61(Suppl 8):43–9.
25. Rogers C. On becoming a person. New edition; 2004.
26. Bowers L, Brennan G, Winship G, Theodoridou C. How expert nurses communicate with acutely psychotic patients. Ment Health Pract. 2010;13(7):24–6.
27. Pritchard JC, Brighty A. Caring for older people experiencing agitation. Nurs Stand. 2015;29(30):49–58.
28. Morandi A, Brummel N, Ely E. Sedation, delirium and mechanical ventilation: the 'ABCDEF' approach. Curr Opin Crit Care. 2011;17(1):43–9.
29. Basten CJ, McGuire BE. Delirium: the role of the psychologist in assessment and management. Aust Psychol. 2011;35(3):201–7.
30. Scottish Intercollegiate Guidelines Network (SIGN) 157. Risk reduction and management of delirium. Edinburgh: SIGN; 2019. 47 p.
31. Girard TD, Exline MC, Carson SS, Hough CL, Rock P, Gong MN, et al. Haloperidol and ziprasidone for treatment of delirium in critical illness. N Engl J Med. 2018;379:2506–16.
32. Bannon L, McGaughey J, Verghis R, Clarke M, McAuley DF, Blackwood B. The effectiveness of non-pharmacological interventions in reducing the incidence and duration of delirium in critically ill patients: a systematic review and meta-analysis. Intensive Care Med. 2019;45(1):1–12.
33. National Institute for Health and Care Excellence. Rehabilitation after critical illness in adults: clinical guideline 83. 2009. https://www.nice.org.uk/guidance/cg83. Accessed 29 Sep 2019.
34. National Institute for Health and Care Excellence. Rehabilitation after critical illness in adults: NICE Quality Standard 158. 2017. https://www.nice.org.uk/guidance/qs158/resources/rehabilitation-after-critical-illness-in-adults-pdf-75545546693317. Accessed 29 Sep 2019.
35. The Faculty of Intensive Care Medicine. Guidelines for the provision of intensive care services. Edition 2. 2019. https://www.ficm.ac.uk/sites/default/files/gpics-v2.pdf. Accessed 29 Sep 2019.

36. Birk JL, Sumner JA, Haerizadeh M, Heyman-Kantor R, Falzon L, Gonzalez C, et al. Early interventions to prevent post-traumatic stress disorder symptoms in survivors of life-threatening medical events: a systematic review. J Anxiety Disord. 2019;64:24–39.
37. Wade DF, Moon Z, Windgassen SS, Harrison AM, Morris L, Weinman JA. Non-pharmacological interventions to reduce ICU-related psychological distress: a systematic review. Minerva Anestesiol. 2016;82(4):465–78.
38. Peris A, Bonizzoli M, Iozzelli D, Migliaccio ML, Zagli G, Bacchereti A, et al. Early intra-intensive care unit psychological intervention promotes recovery from post-traumatic stress disorders, anxiety and depression symptoms in critically ill patients. Crit Care. 2011;15(1):R41.
39. Bryant RA. Acute stress disorder. Curr Opin Psychol. 2017;14:127–31.
40. National Institute for Health and Care Excellence. Post-traumatic stress disorder: NICE guideline 116. 2018. https://www.nice.org.uk/guidance/ng116/chapter/Recommendations#management-of-ptsd-in-children-young-people-and-adults. Accessed 29 Sep 2019.
41. WHO. Psychological first aid; guide for field workers. 2011. https://www.who.int/mental_health/publications/guide_field_workers/en/. Accessed 29 Sep 2019.
42. Wade DM, Mouncey PR, Richards-Belle A, Wulff J, Harrison DA, Sadique MZ, et al. Effect of a nurse-led preventive psychological intervention on symptoms of post-traumatic stress disorder among critically ill patients: a randomised clinical trial. JAMA. 2019;321(7):665–75.
43. Fowler D, Garety P, Kuipers E. Cognitive behaviour therapy for psychosis: theory and practice. Chichester: Wiley; 1995.
44. Mouncey PR, Wade D, Richards-Belle A, Sadique Z, Wulff J, Grieve R, et al. A nurse-led, preventive, psychological intervention to reduce PTSD symptom severity in critically ill patients: the POPPI feasibility study and cluster RCT. Health Serv Deliv Res. 2019;7(30):1.
45. Bennun I. Intensive care unit syndrome: a consideration of psychological interventions. Br J Med Psychol. 2001;74(3):369–77.
46. Varga K, Varga Z, Frituz G. Psychological support based on positive suggestions in the treatment of a critically ill ICU patient—a case report. Interv Med Appl Sci. 2013;5(4):153–61.
47. Sideris T. From post-traumatic stress disorder to absolute dependence in an intensive care unit: reflections on a clinical account. Med Humanit. 2019;45(1):37–44.
48. Cohen JN, Gopal A, Roberts KJ, Anderson E, Siegal AM. Ventilator dependent patients successfully weaned with cognitive behavioural therapy: a case series. Psychosomatics. 2019;60:612–9.
49. National Institute for Health and Care Excellence. Depression in adults: recognition and management clinical guideline: NICE guideline [CG90]. 2009. https://www.nice.org.uk/guidance/cg90/resources/depression-in-adults-recognition-and-management-975742636741. Accessed 29 Sep 2019.
50. Brummel NE, Girard TD, Ely EW, Pandharipande PP, Morandi A, Hughes CG. Feasibility and safety of early combined cognitive and physical therapy for critically ill medical and surgical patients: the activity and cognitive therapy in ICU (ACT-ICU) trial. Intensive Care Med. 2014;40(3):370–9.
51. Lee HW, Park Y, Jang EJ, Lee YL. Intensive care unit length of stay is reduced by protocolised family support intervention: a systematic review and meta-analysis. Intensive Care Med. 2019;45(8):1072–81.
52. Rosa RG, Falavigna M, da Silva DB, Sganzerla D, Martins M, Santos S, et al. Effect of flexible family visitation on delirium among patients in the intensive care unit. JAMA. 2019;322(3):216–28.
53. Bench S, Day T, Heelas K, Hopkins P, White C, Griffiths P. Evaluating the feasibility and effectiveness of a critical care discharge information pack for patients and their families: a pilot cluster randomised controlled trial. BMJ Open. 2015;5(11):e006852.
54. Cuthbertson BH, Rattray J, Campbell MK, Gager M, Roughton S, Smith A, et al. The PRaCTICaL study of nurse led, intensive care follow-up programmes for improving long term outcomes from critical illness: a pragmatic randomised controlled trial. BMJ. 2009;339:b3723.

55. Schofield-Robinson O, Lewis SR, Smith AF, McPeake J, Alderton P. Follow-up services for improving long-term outcomes in intensive care unit (ICU) survivors. Cochrane Database Syst Rev. 2018;11(11):CD012701.
56. Girbes AR, Beishuizen A. Interfacing the ICU with the general practitioner. Crit Care. 2010;14(3):172.
57. McPeake J, Shaw M, Iwashyna TJ, Daniel M, Devine H, Jarvie L, et al. Intensive care syndrome: promoting independence and return to employment (InS:PIRE). Early evaluation of a complex intervention. PLoS One. 2017;12(11):e0188028.
58. Griffiths RD, Jones C. Filling the intensive care memory gap? Intensive Care Med. 2001;27(2):344–6.
59. Garrouste-Orgeas M, Flahault C, Vinatier I, Rigaud JP, Thieulot-Rolin N, Mercier E, et al. Effect of an ICU diary on post-traumatic stress disorder symptoms among patients receiving mechanical ventilation: a randomised clinical trial. JAMA. 2019;322(3):229–39.
60. Aitkin LM, Rattray J, Kenardy J, Hull AM, Ullman AJ, Brocque L, et al. Perspectives of patients and family members regarding intensive care diaries: an exploratory mixed methods study. J Crit Care. 2017;38:263–8.
61. McPeake J, Hirshberg EL, Christie LM, Drumright K, Haines K, Hough CL, et al. Models of peer support to remediate post-intensive care syndrome: a report developed by the Society of Critical Care Medicine Thrive International Peer Support Collaborative. Crit Care Med. 2019;47(1):e21–7.
62. Theikling. Support groups for 'ICU survivors' are springing up. But will patients traumatised by intensive care show up? Stat News. 2017. https://www.statnews.com/2017/07/24/icu-patient-support-group/.
63. Haines KJ, Sevin CM, Hibbert E, Boehm LM, Aparanji K, Bakhru RN, et al. Key mechanisms by which post-ICU activities can improve in-ICU care: results of the international THRIVE collaboratives. Intensive Care Med. 2019;45(7):939–47.
64. Jensen JF, Egerod I, Bestle MH, Christensen DF, Elklit A, Hansen RL, et al. A recovery program to improve quality of life, sense of coherence and psychological health in ICU survivors: a multicenter randomised controlled trial, the RAPIT study. Intensive Care Med. 2016;42:1733–43.
65. Cox CE, Hough CL, Jones DM, Ungar A, Reagan W, Key MD, et al. Effects of mindfulness training programmes delivered by a self-directed mobile app and by telephone compared with an education programme for survivors of critical illness: a pilot randomised clinical trial. Thorax. 2018;74(1):33–42.
66. Cox CE, Hough CL, Carson SS, White DB, Kahn JM, Olsen MK, et al. Effects of a telephone- and web-based coping skills training program compared with an education program for survivors of critical illness and their family members. A randomised clinical trial. Am J Respir Crit Care Med. 2018;197:66–78.
67. Brewin CR, Rumball F, Happé F. Neglected causes of post-traumatic stress disorder. BMJ. 2019;10:365.
68. Hulme T. Using eye movement therapy to reduce trauma after intensive care. Nurs Times. 2018;114(3):18–21.
69. Bates A, Golding H, Rushbrook S, Shapiro E, Pattison N, Baldwin D, et al. A randomised pilot feasibility study of eye movement desensitisation and reprocessing recent traumatic episode protocol, to improve psychological recovery following intensive care admission for COVID-19. JICS. 2022;24:309.
70. National Institute for Health and Care Excellence. Generalised anxiety disorder and panic disorder in adults: management. Clinical guideline 113. 2019. https://www.nice.org.uk/guidance/cg113. Accessed 29 Sep 2019.
71. Jackson JC, Ely EW, Morey MC, Anderson VM, Denne LB, Clune J, et al. Cognitive and physical rehabilitation of intensive care unit survivors: results of the RETURN randomised controlled pilot investigation. Crit Care Med. 2012;40(4):1088–97.
72. Wilson JE, Collar EM, Kiehl AL, Lee H, Merzenich M, Ely EW, et al. Computerised cognitive rehabilitation in intensive care unit survivors: returning to everyday tasks using reha-

bilitation networks-computerised cognitive rehabilitation pilot investigation. Ann Am Thorac Soc. 2018;15(7):887–91.

73. Wang S, Hammes J, Khan S, Gao S, Harrawood A, Martinez S, et al. Improving recovery and outcomes every day after the ICU (IMPROVE): study protocol for a randomised controlled trial. Trials. 2018;19(1):196.

74. Ley H, Skorniewska Z, Harrison PJ, Taquet M. Risks of neurological and psychiatric sequelae 2 years after hospitalisation or admission to ICU for COVID-19 compared to admissions for other causes. Brain Behav Immunity. 2023;112:85–95.

75. Greenberg N, Weston D, Hall C, Caulfield T, Williamson V, Fong K. Mental health of staff working in intensive care during Covid-19. Occup Med. 2021;71:62–7.

76. Colville GA, Smith JG, Brierley J, Citron K, Nguru NM, Shaunak PD, et al. Coping with staff burnout and work-related posttraumatic stress in intensive care. Paediatr Crit Care Med. 2017;18:e267–73.

77. Beadman M, Highfield J, Wade D, et al. The health of intensive care unit teams: moving beyond a trauma focus. Occup Med. 2021;71(8):386–7.

78. Hall CE, Milward J, Spoiala C, Bhogal JK, Weston D, Potts HWW, et al. The mental health of staff working on intensive care units over the COVID-19 winter surge of 2020 in England: a cross sectional survey. Br J Anaesth. 2022;128:971–9.

Post-intensive Care Syndrome

11

Ramona O. Hopkins and David McWilliams

11.1 A History of PICS

In the 1990s, increasing interest around the long-term impact of Acute Respiratory Distress Syndrome (ARDS) led to the consideration of longer term outcomes. These early questions centred around the concept that a patient survives, but what happens to the lungs after ARDS? Do they recover or are they irreparably damaged as a consequence of ARDS and the associated need for prolonged invasive ventilation? With an early focus on pulmonary function, several studies identified residual impairments in lung diffusion capacity and the presence of restrictive or obstructive impairments [1, 2]. This increased interest in the wider implications of this pulmonary dysfunction, and a study by McHugh and colleagues found that not only did ARDS survivors have pulmonary impairments, but they also had health complaints, had not returned to their normal function and less than half had returned to work at 1 year [3]. Aside from the physical impact, a subsequent landmark study in 1999 assessed cognitive function, health related quality of life, and mental health (depression and anxiety) in ARDS survivors 1 year after hospital discharge [4]. This study found cognitive impairments were present in 100% of survivors at hospital discharge, with 30% still demonstrating impairments in attention, memory, processing speed and global cognitive decline 1 year after discharge from hospital. Further to this, survivors were found to have a multitude of other problems including reduced

R. O. Hopkins (✉)
Psychology Department and Neuroscience Center, Brigham Young University, Provo, UT, USA
e-mail: ramona_hopkins@byu.edu

D. McWilliams
Centre for Care Excellence, Coventry University, Coventry, UK
e-mail: david.mcwilliams@uhcw.nhs.uk

quality of life, bodily pain, fatigue and ongoing physical problems. As a result, many had not resumed their normal activities or returned to work at 1 year.

Increased recognition of the longer term impact of critical illness and or its treatment on a variety of body systems served as a stark warning to clinicians that survival alone was insufficient when evaluating patient outcomes. This led to an increased focus on the evaluation of longer term physical and neuromuscular outcomes [5] along with greater consideration of the potential for long-term psychological impacts [6]. For example, Herridge and colleagues assessed 109 ARDS survivors at 3, 6 and 12 months and found abnormalities in pulmonary function, impaired health related quality of life and a reduced distance walked in 6 min at all three time points [7]. Importantly, whilst the distance walked improved over time, it failed to reach predicted distances observed for age matched healthy subjects, and was still only around two thirds of what would be expected at 1 year following hospital discharge.

As the research on outcomes after critical illness continued to expand, questions remained as to whether these adverse outcomes subsequently improved after a year, or whether they continued to persist over time. In 2005, Hopkins and colleagues found cognitive impairments remained even 2 years after leaving the hospital, with 80% of patients having cognitive impairments at hospital discharge, 45% at 1 year and 44% at 2 years [8]. Rather than continuing to improve, from a cognitive perspective at least recovery appeared to plateau at 1 year, with minimal to no change after this time point. Similarly, ongoing work by Herridge and colleagues in 2005 found that ARDS survivors continued to have functional limitations, with no further improvement in the distance walked in 6 min at 2 years, coupled with an apparent further reduction in their quality of life over the same time period [9]. Also at 2 years, only around two thirds of survivors had returned to work, with those who had not returned suffering with depression, post-traumatic stress disorder, muscle weakness, fatigue, and cognitive impairments. These and other findings of persistent adverse long-term outcomes highlighted an urgent need to identify possible interventions to improve outcomes, strategies to prevent or minimise negative outcomes and the need to develop organised targeted follow-up for survivors of critical illness.

The landmark 2002 Report from the Brussels Roundtable was one of the first meetings which addressed the long-term outcomes following critical illness. Notably the report highlighted the consideration of patient survivorship, specifically asking the question of what this survival really means and whether ICU care decisions would change if more was known about these patient related outcomes [10]. This meeting assessed research to date, causes and modifiers of long-term outcomes, and discussed the future for both clinical care and research for improved care. The report proposed recommendations for future research including observational studies of long-term outcomes, studies that assessed outcomes and burden of family and informal caregivers, long-term economic costs of adverse outcomes, and interventional trials to better understand how outcomes could be prevented or improved [10]. Predominantly though, the Brussels Round Table was a resounding call to focus on how critical illness and its treatments affects patients and families.

As outcomes research increased, several gaps in the literature were found with little consensus or information to guide measuring outcomes, properties of the measurement tools, timing of outcomes assessment, which outcome domains should be assessed, or exposures in the ICU that may contribute to long-term outcomes to mention a few. In addition, there was a paucity of information or guidance on which aspects of critical illness were important in determining long-term outcomes. To address these gaps, Needham and colleagues developed recommendations on potential outcomes and exposure variables for use in long-term outcomes research [11]. This was an important foundation on which to develop and improve outcomes research. Groups were categorised to include the following.

11.2   Outcomes

1. Medical outcomes, such as survival, new diagnoses and hospital readmission.
2. Patient outcomes such as impairment and disability, functional status and quality of life.
3. Caregiver outcomes, such as anxiety, depression or post-traumatic stress disorder.

11.3   Exposures

(a) Patient-based exposures such as demographic information and diagnosis.
(b) Clinical management exposures, such as medications and procedures.
(c) ICU organisational exposures, such as staffing of physicians and nurses, hospital teaching, use of clinical protocols and teamwork factors.

11.4   Defining Post-intensive Care Syndrome

In 2010 the Society of Critical Care Medicine held a stakeholder meeting to improve long-term outcomes after critical illness [12]. The meeting consisted of 31 invited international experts and stakeholders. A key goal of the meeting was to raise awareness of the issue by developing and agreeing on the term 'Post-Intensive Care Syndrome' to describe the observed long-term impairment after critical illness for both patients and families. Post-intensive care syndrome was described as new or worsening impairment in physical, cognitive or mental health after critical illness persisting beyond the acute care period. A major goal of the stakeholders meeting was to improve awareness and education leading to improved screening and to prompt research [12]. Importantly, it was acknowledged that due to the diverse nature of PICS, in which an unspecified number of impairments across three domains (mental health, cognitive impairments and physical impairments), no one clear diagnostic test or tool should be used to determine if someone has PICS or not. Instead, it was recommended that PICS should be considered as a framework to evaluate multiple aspects of recovery. The management of PICS would therefore require collaboration between practitioners and researchers in both inpatient and community settings to improve care for survivors and their families.

A second Society of Critical Care stakeholders meeting was held in 2012 which included broader representation of professional associations and health systems involved in rehabilitation of ICU survivors [13]. The goal of the task force was to increase awareness and develop programmes of education to increase widespread understanding of post intensive care syndrome, and develop an action plan (including research areas) with a goal of improving patient and family outcomes. This meeting emphasised the need for systematic recognition of mental health, cognitive, and/or physical impairments related to post intensive care syndrome and the need for targeted research to develop tools to assess outcomes, understand the mechanisms and risk factors for the development of PICS and ultimately to evaluate potential interventions.

As understanding around PICS improved, new approaches to classification have been proposed. A study by Brown and colleagues in 2017 [14] identified four unique subtypes of PICS including patients with:

1. Mild impairments in physical and mental health.
2. Moderate impairments physical and mental health.
3. Moderate impairment in mental health and severe impairments in physical health.
4. Severe impairments in both physical and mental health.

It is unclear if these subtypes will be replicated in other studies, but what may be the case is that these different groups may require targeted treatments to address their unique presentations of PICS. Specifically, the authors proposed these subtypes may help direct the development of tailored rehabilitation strategies, including investigations of combined physical and mental health interventions, and distinct interventions to improve cognitive outcomes.

A review in 2021 that assessed long-term outcomes after critical illness proposed expanding the 'definition' of post-intensive care syndrome to include functional disabilities, osteopenia, metabolic disorder, endocrine dysfunction, vulnerability, fatigue, sleep disorders and pain [15]. This raises the question whether disorders with long-term effects such as osteopenia, metabolic disorder and endocrine dysfunction be included as part of PICS? Other disorders such as chronic pain, sleep and fatigue could be included under physical impairment. However, the term Post Intensive Care Syndrome was adopted principally to raise awareness, improve education about adverse long-term outcomes and NOT to act as a diagnostic classification. Moreover, Rousseau et al., 2021 suggest PICS be used as an umbrella term rather than a set of well-defined and researched outcomes [15]. The question this raises is whether every new condition that is identified should be included as part of PICS? For example, should new onset diabetes [16] be included in the definition of PICS or instead be viewed as another post-ICU medical condition or exacerbation of an underlying medical problem. What can be considered as a consequence of critical illness, and what would be considered as a worsening of the underlying medical condition. The complex interaction between consequences of a critical illness and a worsening of the underlying medical condition requires careful consideration. The key message remains regarding the need for holistic, patient centred approaches to care, both for assessment of rehabilitation need and the delivery of individualised rehabilitation interventions.

11.5   Diagnosis and Assessment of PICS

There exists a lack of agreement on which instruments should be used to assess PICS, and how frequently assessment should take place. Subsequently, there is no single test or diagnostic tool specifically designed to diagnose PICS [17]. As PICS encompasses a broad range of physical, cognitive, and psychological impairments, current diagnostics approaches involve each component to be identified and addressed separately [18]. A collaborative approach for patients recovering from critical illness to include healthcare professionals from various disciplines is essential to avoid unmet rehabilitation needs. This may include including intensivists, rehabilitation specialists, nurses, physiotherapists, occupational therapists, dietitians, speech and language therapist and mental health professionals. This interdisciplinary approach allows for a comprehensive assessment and management plan tailored to the individual's needs [18].

It's important to recognise that PICS is a complex and multifaceted condition, and diagnosis requires careful consideration of the patient's medical history, clinical presentation and functional status. A thorough clinical assessment is required, where healthcare providers conduct a thorough medical history and physical examination to assess the patient's overall health and identify any physical or cognitive impairment. This may include evaluating muscle strength, mobility, balance and coordination, as well as assessing cognitive function, memory, attention and executive functioning. Functional assessments should also be performed to evaluate the patient's ability to perform activities of daily living (ADLs) and instrumental activities of daily living (IADLs) [19]. These assessments help identify any limitations in functional independence and guide rehabilitation planning. Consideration should also be made to the assessment of non-physical aspects of recovery, psychological evaluation assesses the presence of symptoms such as anxiety, depression, posttraumatic stress disorder (PTSD), cognitive impairments and insomnia. This evaluation may involve standardised psychological assessments, clinical interviews and self-report questionnaires.

11.6   Screening Tools

As discussed above, a variety of screening tools and questionnaires may be used to assess specific individual aspects of PICS, such as physical function, cognitive function and psychological symptoms. More recently, attempts have been made to develop core outcome sets aiming to both standardise diagnosis, as well as ensuring consistency in research outcomes evaluated. Spies et al. [20] used a three round consensus approach to evaluate instruments for use in outpatient settings in survivors of critical illness. They recommended a two-step approach that uses both questionnaires and performance-based measures, first screening and then in-depth assessment [20].

Further interest in this area spiked after the COVID-19 pandemic, with large numbers of patients admitted to critical care meaning unprecedented numbers of patients surviving critical illness being left with significant physical and psychological morbidity. The Post Intensive Care Unit Presentation Screen (PICUPS) tool [21], developed by the United Kingdom Intensive Care Societies National Rehabilitation Collaborative, is one such multidimensional tool with the aim to identify post intensive care syndrome. The PICUPS tool has been demonstrated as an effective screening tool for PICS highlighting potential rehabilitation needs, which may have been missed by clinical opinion alone. This subsequently triggers referrals for more specialist assessment and treatment.

11.7   Prevalence and Features of PICS

A major feature of PICS and corresponding physical dysfunction is related to ICU-acquired weakness (ICU-AW), which is defined as muscle weakness which develops during an ICU stay. This is a common problem of being critically ill and occurs in 30–50% of patients admitted to ICU [22]. ICU-AW makes the activities of daily living difficult, including grooming, dressing, feeding, bathing and walking for up to a year post hospital discharge [23]. Around a third of patients still require help with at least one activity of daily living and less than half returning to work 1 year following hospital discharge [24].

Following hospital discharge, 30–80% of critical care survivors may experience cognitive or brain dysfunction [25, 26]. This often presents as problems with memory, concentration, problem solving and organising and working on complex tasks. Cognitive impairments may affect whether the patient can return to work, balance a checkbook or perform other tasks that involve organisation and concentration. Other mental health problems are also common with PICS. Critical care survivors may develop problems with falling or staying asleep. They may have nightmares and unwanted memories. Reminders of their illness may produce intense feelings or strong, clear images in their mind. Their reactions to these feelings may be physical or emotional and up to one in five may have symptoms of post-traumatic stress disorder [27]. These include having nightmares and unwanted memories, and wanting to avoid thinking or talking about their stay in the ICU.

11.8   PICS-F

Recognition of the significant impact of critical illness on families and relatives has led to the expansion of the categorisation of PICS to include Post-Intensive Care Syndrome Family (PICS-F). PICS-F refers to the impact that critical illness and

ICU experience can have on their family members or caregivers. Just as patients who survive critical illness in the ICU may experience physical, cognitive and psychological impairments, their family members may also experience a range of emotional, psychological and social challenges [28, 29].

Family members of ICU patients often undergo significant stress, anxiety and emotional burden during the patient's critical illness and recovery process. They may experience feelings of helplessness, fear, guilt and grief. Additionally, the practical demands of caregiving and navigating the complex healthcare system can contribute to their stress and emotional strain.

PICS-F highlights the importance of recognizing and addressing the needs of family members and caregivers of ICU patients, both during the patient's ICU stay and after discharge. Providing support, education and resources to family members can help them cope with the challenges they face and improve their ability to support the patient's recovery process. This may include providing access to counseling services, support groups and educational materials about critical illness and recovery.

11.9 Conclusion

Patients surviving a period of critical illness are often left with significant physical, mental and emotional sequelae. These problems can persist for months or even years, and recovery is often incomplete. Over the last two decades, much has been learned about the scale and impact of this post intensive care syndrome, with early management within the ICU essential to improve outcomes. The following chapters will explore the key components of holistic, multi-professional care to improve outcomes and support recovery.

References

1. Elliott CG, Rasmusson BY, Crapo RO, Morris AH, Jensen RL. Prediction of pulmonary function abnormalities after adult respiratory distress syndrome (ARDS). Am Rev Respir Dis. 1987;135(3):634–8.
2. Peters JI, Bell RC, Prihoda TJ, et al. Clinical determinants of abnormalities in pulmonary functions in survivors of the adult respiratory distress syndrome. Am Rev Respir Dis. 1989;139(5):1163–8.
3. McHugh LG, Milberg JA, Whitcomb ME, et al. Recovery of function in survivors of the acute respiratory distress syndrome. Am J Respir Crit Care Med. 1994;150(1):90–4.
4. Hopkins RO, Weaver LK, Pope D, Orme JF, Bigler ED, Larson-LOHR V. Neuropsychological sequelae and impaired health status in survivors of severe acute respiratory distress syndrome. Am J Respir Crit Care Med. 1999;160(1):50–6.
5. Fletcher SN, Kennedy DD, Ghosh IR, Misra VP, Kiff K, Coakley JH, Hinds CJ. Persistent neuromuscular and neurophysiologic abnormalities in long-term survivors of prolonged critical illness. Crit Care Med. 2003;31(4):1012–6.

6. Kress JP, Gehlbach B, Lacy M, Pliskin N, Pohlman AS, Hall JB. The long-term psychological effects of daily sedative interruption on critically ill patients. Am J Respir Crit Care Med.
   2003;168(12):1457–61.
7. Herridge MS, Cheung AM, Tansey CM, Matte-Martyn A, Diaz-Granados N, Al-Saidi
   F, Cooper AB, Guest CB, Mazer CD, Mehta S, Stewart TE, Barr A, Cook D, Slutsky AS,
   Canadian Critical Care Trials Group. One-year outcomes in survivors of the acute respiratory
   distress syndrome. N Engl J Med. 2003;348(8):683–93.
8. Hopkins RO, Weaver LK, Collingridge D, Parkinson RB, Chan KJ, Orme JF Jr. Two-year
   cognitive, emotional, and quality-of-life outcomes in acute respiratory distress syndrome. Am
   J Respir Crit Care Med. 2005;171(4):340–7.
9. Cheung AM, Tansey CM, Tomlinson G, Diaz-Granados N, Matté A, Barr A, Mehta S, Mazer
   CD, Guest CB, Stewart TE, Al-Saidi F, Cooper AB, Cook D, Slutsky AS, Herridge MS. Two-
   year outcomes, health care use, and costs of survivors of acute respiratory distress syndrome.
   Am J Respir Crit Care Med. 2006;174(5):538–44.
10. Angus DC, Carlet J, 2002 Brussels Roundtable Participants. Surviving intensive care: a report
    from the 2002 Brussels Roundtable. Intensive Care Med. 2003;29(3):368–77.
11. Needham DM, Dowdy DW, Mendez-Tellez PA, Herridge MS, Pronovost PJ. Studying out-
    comes of intensive care unit survivors: measuring exposures and outcomes. Intensive Care
    Med. 2005;31(9):1153–60.
12. Needham DM, Davidson J, Cohen H, Hopkins RO, Weinert C, Wunsch H, Zawistowski C,
    Bemis-Dougherty A, Berney SC, Bienvenu OJ, Brady SL, Brodsky MB, Denehy L, Elliott
    D, Flatley C, Harabin AL, Jones C, Louis D, Meltzer W, Muldoon SR, Palmer JB, Perme
    C, Robinson M, Schmidt DM, Scruth E, Spill GR, Storey CP, Render M, Votto J, Harvey
    MA. Improving long-term outcomes after discharge from intensive care unit: report from a
    stakeholders' conference. Crit Care Med. 2012;40(2):502–9.
13. Elliott D, Davidson JE, Harvey MA, Bemis-Dougherty A, Hopkins RO, Iwashyna TJ, Wagner
    J, Weinert C, Wunsch H, Bienvenu OJ, Black G, Brady S, Brodsky MB, Deutschman C, Doepp
    D, Flatley C, Fosnight S, Gittler M, Gomez BT, Hyzy R, Louis D, Mandel R, Maxwell C,
    Muldoon SR, Perme CS, Reilly C, Robinson MR, Rubin E, Schmidt DM, Schuller J, Scruth E,
    Siegal E, Spill GR, Sprenger S, Straumanis JP, Sutton P, Swoboda SM, Twaddle ML, Needham
    DM. Exploring the scope of post-intensive care syndrome therapy and care: engagement of
    non-critical care providers and survivors in a second stakeholders meeting. Crit Care Med.
    2014;42(12):2518–26.
14. Brown SM, Wilson EL, Presson AP, Dinglas VD, Greene T, Hopkins RO, Needham DM, with
    the National Institutes of Health NHLBI ARDS Network. Understanding patient outcomes
    after acute respiratory distress syndrome: identifying subtypes of physical, cognitive and men-
    tal health outcomes. Thorax. 2017;72(12):1094–103.
15. Rousseau AF, Prescott HC, Brett SJ, Weiss B, Azoulay E, Creteur J, Latronico N, Hough CL,
    Weber-Carstens S, Vincent JL, Preiser JC. Long-term outcomes after critical illness: recent
    insights. Crit Care. 2021;25(1):108.
16. Ali Abdelhamid Y, Kar P, Finnis ME, et al. Stress hyperglycaemia in critically ill patients and
    the subsequent risk of diabetes: a systematic review and meta-analysis. Crit Care. 2016;20:301.
    https://doi.org/10.1186/s13054-016-1471-6.
17. Berger P, Braude D. Post-intensive care syndrome: screening and management in primary care.
    Aust J Gen Pract. 2021;50(10):737–40. https://doi.org/10.31128/AJGP-07-20-55492. PMID:
    34590093.
18. Iwashyna TJ, Netzer G. The burdens of survivorship: an approach to thinking about long-term
    outcomes after critical illness. Semin Respir Crit Care Med. 2012;33(4):327–38.
19. Hopkins RO, Suchyta MR, Kamdar BB, Darowski E, Jackson JC, Needham DM. Instrumental
    activities of daily living after critical illness: a systematic review. Ann Am Thorac Soc.
    2017;14(8):1332–43.
20. Spies CD, Krampe H, Paul N, Denke C, Kiselev J, Piper SK, Kruppa J, Grunow JJ, Steinecke
    K, Gülmez T, Scholtz K, Rosseau S, Hartog C, Busse R, Caumanns J, Marschall U, Gersch
    M, Apfelbacher C, Weber-Carstens S, Weiss B. Instruments to measure outcomes of post-

intensive care syndrome in outpatient care settings—results of an expert consensus and feasibility field test. J Intensive Care Soc. 2021;22(2):159–74.
21. Puthucheary Z, Brown C, Corner E, Wallace S, Highfield J, Bear D, Rehill N, Montgomery H, Aitken L, Turner-Stokes L. The post-ICU presentation screen (PICUPS) and rehabilitation prescription (RP) for intensive care survivors part II: clinical engagement and future directions for the national Post-Intensive care Rehabilitation Collaborative. J Intensive Care Soc. 2022;23(3):264–72.
22. Fan E, Cheek F, Chlan L, et al. An official American Thoracic Society Clinical Practice guideline: the diagnosis of intensive care unit-acquired weakness in adults. Am J Respir Crit Care Med. 2014;190:1437–46.
23. Hermans G, Van Mechelen H, Clerckx B, Vanhullebusch T, Mesotten D, Wilmer A, et al. Acute outcomes and 1-year mortality of intensive care unit-acquired weakness: a cohort study and propensity-matched analysis. Am J Respir Crit Care Med. 2014;190:410–20.
24. Batchelor A. Getting it right first time—adult critical care; 2021.
25. Harvey MA, Davidson JE. Post-intensive care syndrome: right care, right now…and later. Crit Care Med. 2016;44:381–5.
26. Pandharipande PP, Girard TD, Jackson JC, et al. Long-term cognitive impairment after critical illness. N Engl J Med. 2013;369:1306–16.
27. Griffiths J, Hatch RA, Bishop J, et al. An exploration of social and economic outcome and associated health-related quality of life after critical illness in general intensive care unit survivors: a 12-month follow-up study. Crit Care. 2013;17:R100.
28. van den Born-van Zanten SA, Dongelmans DA, Dettling-Ihnenfeldt D, Vink R, van der Schaaf M. Caregiver strain and posttraumatic stress symptoms of informal caregivers of intensive care unit survivors. Rehabil Psychol. 2016;61(2):173–8.
29. Wintermann GB, Weidner K, Strauß B, Rosendahl J, Petrowski K. Predictors of posttraumatic stress and quality of life in family members of chronically critically ill patients after intensive care. Ann Intensive Care. 2016;6(1):69.

End-of-Life Care: A Dignified Death

12

Julie Benbenishty

This chapter explores multi-dimensional end-of-life care in critical care settings. Typically, patients are admitted to intensive care with the aim to achieve curative goals of care and hopes of recovery. A patient can quickly deteriorate, and the transition from critical illness to the point of futility and the processes of dying may be rapid and difficult to manage [1]. One of the greatest challenges across health care teams continues to be consensus and acceptance of the concept of futility of treatment and the concept of dying [2].

Critical care teams identify decision-making regarding goals of care are sensitive to multiple and often changing parameters. These include fluctuating responses to treatments, preferences of families which may change over time, coupled with the perceptions and opinions of the multi professional team. In the normal course of critical care, recognition that curative interventions where goals of treatment are not being effective, should stimulate ICU professionals to explore other approaches in order to preserve dignity while providing holistic care.

For the 20% of ICU patients who die in the ICU, there is a need to focus on transition from curative interventions to end-of-life care (EOLC), rather than end-of-life care itself assuring effective and timely decision making underpins their care [2]. In intensive care settings, it is acknowledged this transition from curative intervention to end of life (EOL) is often a complex process, with many decisive turning points at which decisions must be made and actions taken. A phased transition, or simultaneous care approach, recognises treatment goals evolve and perhaps becomes particularly relevant for patients with non-cancer conditions, where the trajectory of decline may be both unpredictable and highly variable. Although EOL

J. Benbenishty (✉)
Hebrew University Faculty of Medicine School of Nursing, Jerusalem, Israel
e-mail: julie@hadassah.org.il

181

C. Boulanger, D. McWilliams (eds.), *Passport to Successful Outcomes for Patients Admitted to ICU*, https://doi.org/10.1007/978-3-031-53019-7_12

recommendations for critically ill patients exist [3], the actual development of a clear pathway for end-of-life care in clinical practice is recognised as complex [4]. Nurses can however use a set of competencies or care bundles to guide care during the transition phase and throughout these decisive turning points.

A care bundle identifies a set of key interventions often derived from evidence-based guidelines which when implemented, are expected to improve patients' health outcomes [5]. Care bundles are used to implement behavior change in ICU and can lead to standardised care, ultimately improving outcomes and staff satisfaction [6]. Decisive turning points are defined as 'relatively short periods of time during which there is a substantially heightened probability that agents' choices will affect the outcome of interest' [7]. Capoccia's study of decisive turning points identified the necessity for appropriate communication during critical events. Events such as the first visit of the family to ICU, moving a dying patient to a ward or the first discussion with a consultant which can make or break the family's willingness to accept that the patient may die. Examples such as 'doctors will sometimes say "well they may not get better" or "they're unlikely to improve" when actually the patient is going to die' [7]. Decisive turning points are used as a timeline for the clinician to consider what needs to be accomplished or addressed during the transition period. Hence, they are prompts rather than recommendations.

Today's challenge for ICU clinicians is to understand and implement patient/ family centred end-of-life wishes. By understanding scientifically based decisive turning points a systematic approach to transition can be adopted, from curative interventions to end-of-life measures. This chapter aims to synthesise theories, interventional studies and accepted guidelines into a methodological strategy of end-of-life care processes. The next step is to intervene to stabilise the family/ patient crisis through cultural, ethical, spiritual and therapeutic targeted communication. In this journey, we incorporate interventions supporting grief, bereavement and follow-up care. The following model offers a care bundle.

12.1   Components of the Theoretical Model

Today's challenge for ICU clinicians is to understand and implement patient/family centred end-of-life wishes. Understanding these decisive turning points together with relevant supporting literature, a systematic approach to transition from curative interventions to end-of-life measures can be implemented. The aim of this integrated model is synthesising theories, interventional studies and accepted guidelines into a methodological strategy of end-of-life care processes— from identification of the non-responsive patient and assessing life threatening end-of-life conditions, with a focus on collaborative decision making throughout. The next step is to then intervene to stabilise the family/patient crisis through cultural, ethical, spiritual and therapeutic targeted communication. In this journey, interventions supporting grief, bereavement and follow-up care are incorporated.

12.1.1 Decisive Turning Point 1: Time Out

When the health care team identifies the patient is not responding to treatment, decisive turning point 1 is then initiated. This signifies consideration be given to a change in goals of care. Regularly during daily rounds the question should be asked—'is this patient responding to curative interventions?' Identification of patients who will not survive may be a significant challenge in the intensive care unit (ICU) as the patient's condition is often complex [8], and death may be an unexpected development during the care trajectory [9]. Identification may be further compromised by lack of agreement between different disciplines regarding the goals of end-of-life care [8]. Backs' study of patient and family feedback indicates that patients' and families perceive a conversation about goals of care to require disruption of an existing routine, followed by a process of searching and then reconfiguration, rather than a logical decision process. These findings suggest families and patients prefer proactive suggestions about things 'we can do now' and that physicians should suggest goals and plans [9].

Enabling nurses to identify characteristics of patients not responding to curative interventions and the chances for survival is an important step in reassessment of treatment goals and propose a stock take or Time Out.

12.1.2 Decisive Turning Point 2: Shared Decision-Making

The aim at this decisive turning point is empathetic, full team investment in gaining family, team and if possible patient involvement in decision making on transition of goals of care. Focus on family conferences must occur early and as often as possible ideally from the same healthcare providers [10].

During this time, the nursing team has opportunities:

- To listen and respond to family members.
- To acknowledge and address emotions.
- To pursue key principles of medical ethics and end-of-life care.
- To explore patient preferences.
- To compassionately explain to surrogate decision makers and utilise this time to affirm non-abandonment [11].

In order to establish a trustworthy relationship between family and team members, it is essential to assure consistency in communication, this can be achieved by defining roles of ICU team as per the examples below [12, 13].

The physician provides:

- Medical updates to patients' families.
- Guidelines for care.
- Shared medical advice concerning treatment.
- Daily goals and options other than curative care [11].

Nurses provide:

- Daily information to the families and offering opportunity to clarify issues.
- Time for family to verbalise thoughts, values, interpretation of patient's wishes; is present as a non-coercive, nonjudgmental 'sounding board' as families process their thoughts and feeling.
- Reinforcement of goals of care [14] and in cases where communication does not result in team/family/patient consensus, there should be a reassessment of the decision-making process to identify improvement mediator issues.
- The opportunity to sit face to face with disagreeing partners to understand their perceptions.

Nurses use a wide range of skills in decision-making and assisting patients/families in their decision-making [15]. Learning culturally specific assessment tools, addressing moral and ethical dilemmas and conflicts within the family and ICU team is crucial in maintaining dignity in the end-of-life process [16]. Religion and spirituality are fundamental beliefs which when applied may alleviate distress and emotional suffering [17]. These beliefs should be openly addressed, and the nursing approach should be subtle and gentle in application using nonverbal communication strategies, active listening and cultural and spiritual assessment questionnaires [16, 17]. These are just a few of the many multi-variable competencies' nurses need to deliver dignified, holistic end-of-life nursing care [18].

12.1.3 Decisive Turning Point 3: Consensus

Several studies have identified that physicians may not take the time to clearly understand the surrogate decision makers' perception and understanding of the decisions made [11, 19]. When families meet with ICU physicians, they frequently have insufficient time to share their perspectives on the patient's goals and values or express their own concerns. ICU physicians may miss opportunities for an empathic response to emotions, leaving families too distressed to absorb or integrate information needed for surrogate decision-making [11, 19, 20].

In this decisive turning point, it is imperative that the ICU nurse uses assessment skills to ensure clear comprehension [15]. Conflicts exist where patients families insist on care considered inappropriate by the ICU team, and in patients whose families object to care that physicians prefer to provide. Where such conflicts occur, mediation between families and health care team usually secures successful resolution [21].

The opportunity to listen carefully to family members' concerns responding directly to these concerns is a key component of these discussions [15]. The nurse needs to probe the surrogate decision maker to ensure that they comprehend the scope and implications of the end-of-life decision. Whether it be only non-escalation of therapy or withdrawal of interventions, the nurse should take the time to fully explain the complete implication of every decision [15]. Family/patient understanding should be assessed and assure all measures have been exhausted and instruction and guidance to family and patient that transition to end-of-life care does not mean "no care'.

Asking questions like 'tell me what the doctor told you' and 'describe what you understood form what the physician said' has been found to be helpful in this setting [10]. Communication is one of the most important competencies needed in end-of-life care, encompassing significant expertise in communication, from active listening, comprehension, nonverbal to expression of empathy and hope when confronted with death [15]. There are many publications and resources regarding these various types of communication and how important they are in preserving dignity during nursing end-of-life care [19, 21]. Effective communication in nurse handover is paramount in the continuum of care [12]. Many of the published studies repeatedly show family dissatisfaction with ICU care due to varied messages being delivered by different clinicians, ultimately leading to confusion [8]. Miscommunication also leads to distrust and conflict [4]. A missed opportunity by the team to establish trust and engage the family has a significant impact [11]. It is important to note any conflicts within the nurse-physician team should be resolved before approaching the family [13].

12.1.4 Decisive Turning Point 4: Comfort Care

This decisive turning point focuses on providing symptom management and comfort care including frequent turning, washing, mouth and eye care, massage with perfumed lotion, combing and grooming as well as frequent family visits. If the patient is conscious, then emotional and spiritual support is offered [17, 21]. A clergyman may be called, patient choice music can be played and other spiritual customs and rituals can be suggested [22].

Nurses have described how they use their senses to read patients' bodily experiences, their needs for extensive and 'trifling' nursing care and whether their actions had the desired effects [15, 23]. It can be suggested that it is not until nurses can master machinery and procedures that they can focus on patients as human beings and their needs, enabling patients to tolerate the often-afflicting technology on their bodies [19]. Nurses use 'diagnostic therapeutic touch,' which is mainly executed with an intellectual hand, analyses, diagnoses and promotes comfort [15]. Endacott [18] found that most ICU nurses defined 'a good death' as being able to deliver pain free care, closure and maintaining hygiene [18].

Intensive care nurses perceive adequate pain management, agreement between health professionals on decision-making, and facilitating a comfortable environment for patients and families, during the whole end-of-life process as the priorities of care delivery [18]. This bundle component is essential throughout the transition process and becomes paramount in nursing care delivery when curative interventions cease [24]. A qualitative study found patients describe nursing in end-of-life care and caring throughout the transcripts most often in relation to compassion. The connection between compassion and caring was so strong that many participants did not delineate between the two, often substituting 'compassion' for 'care' and 'caring' throughout the interviews [25]. Martins and Basto [26] demonstrated nursing interventions which relieved patient's end-of-life suffering. These interventions were developed through a process that is interactional, dynamic, integral and systematic. The process included nurses who assisted patients in the last hours of life by providing physical comfort, accepting the reality of their condition, supporting the emotional equilibrium, harmonising the environment, and facilitating friends and family presence. Nurses enable final wishes, spiritual and comfort needs [26].

The presence and assurances by the nurse that they would not leave the patient aimed to maintain patients' meaningful relations and feelings of not being abandoned which avert patients' loneliness [17, 27]. The nurses may perceive that a patient's dignity is threatened if they are over-treated, for instance when relatives wanted to prolong life, or when physicians indecisiveness lead to delayed management of life sustaining interventions, when patients are dying [27]. Nurses also highlight loss of dignity for some patients in relation to changes in appearance: Loss of patient control and dignity can be mitigated by treating every patient respectfully as an individual conscious, awake person [18]. To enhance individuality in daily care, relatives can be encouraged to characterise the patient, to give advice, and bring a picture of the patient to remind them about their previous appearance [27]. It is important to note that end-of-life factors rated important among patients included having funeral arrangements made, feeling one's life was complete, not being a burden to family or society, being able to help others, coming to peace with God and praying [17]. Although most ICU patients are not conscious at EOL, these important factors can be implemented by family members with the support of the bedside nurse [28].

12.1.5 Decisive Turning Point 5: Family Care

Directing attention towards the family when their loved one is going through this transition trajectory is imperative for the impending death to be perceived as a quality experience [2]. Therefore, the nurse must perform a family assessment of cultural, emotional, spiritual and physical needs [16]. Careful time should be directed towards ascertaining family expectations and what their hopes might be, whilst providing reassurance to the family and patient that they will not be abandoned. The ICU nurse can also provide explanations and guidance to the family of what they can do for patient and themselves to assure a meaningful closure [17, 29].

Some additional tools have been evaluated to support patients, families and clinicians [10, 12]. A multicentre study in Europe evaluated a diary intervention in which healthcare staff and family members contributed to a handwritten diary recording events and experiences daily during the patient's ICU stay [30]. Another tool included the development of standardised order sets to support clinicians, prepare families, and ensure patient comfort during limitation of life support [30]. A Dutch study found that families were satisfied with the overall quality of death and dying, feeling supported by the ICU caregivers [31]. Where families felt strongly involved in the decision-making process regarding outcome, satisfaction with the quality of end-of-life care was higher [2]. In a US ICU, a structured palliative care program to improve the quality of end-of-life care was integrated into standard care. This intervention was designed to apply to all patients and their families regardless of their prognosis. Implementation of the intervention changed the qualitative nature of physician rounds and practice. Palliative care domains introduced during the study period were:

- Pain.
- Other symptom management.
- Bereavement/family support.
- Goals-of-care discussions.
- Shared decision making.
- Conflict resolution.

Goals-of-care discussion on physician rounds increased from 2% to 39% of patient-days during the intervention period. These findings demonstrate integration of early palliative care alongside an aggressive, disease-focused, curative care can be accomplished in the ICU for patients without change in mortality. Moreover, this has the ability to improve the end-of-life care practice in such patients [10]. During this decisive turning point, the nursing care provided to family members during this sad and stress filled process impacts significantly on overall family and staff satisfaction as well as overall perception of the provision of quality death in the ICU [18].

To improve communication and alleviate family anxiety during this devastating life-threatening crisis, expertise and competencies in emotional intelligence need to be incorporated. The creation of family support groups whilst their loved one is in ICU has shown promise in fulfilling family needs, while at the same time providing nurses with essential knowledge regarding family capabilities [29, 32]. The extensive body of work from qualitative and quantitative family support group interventions shows new possibilities for nurses to implement this change.

12.1.6 Decisive Turning Point 6: Deceased Care

This decisive turning point is the point in time where nurses care for the deceased body. Efstathiou and Walker in their 2014 study found that a good death promotes comfort as a result of therapeutic interventions ensuring the right to physical integrity, preserving a good body image and ensuring dignity [33]. Vigilance, non-abandonment, the presence of composure and providing a meaningful spiritual closure all encompass good quality after death care [17]. Ensuring a good death means above all to promote comfort through care practices that reconcile rationality and sensibility ensuring the dignity of the patient and his family [18]. Nurses must also identify the importance of considering the place of death [moving to a single room], whether the family can be present and aware of what was going to happen, whilst ensuring the dying patient was pain free, and calm [no agitation or fitting] [18, 28, 34].

Nurses should remove monitoring equipment from the patient and family to 'de-intensify' the environment so that the "patient is given back to the family as they came to us" [18]. In this way, the nurse can support a death which best represents what is perceived to be a good death to both professionally and personally [28]. A study of EOL post death nursing practice found that nurses move patients to private rooms for family privacy, to ensure peaceful dignified bedside scene. The nurses focused on enough family time next to the deceased body to accept the new reality. A Norwegian nursing study demonstrates that music might be helpful for nurses during after-death care as well as for the care of the relatives. Including ambient music in an after-death care can help nurses show respect and dignity to the deceased patient [22]. This decisive turning points includes nurse explanation to family regarding death certificate and hospital procedures.

12.1.7 Decisive Turning Point 7: Follow-Up

This decisive turning point focuses on determining how relatives of deceased ICU patients experienced the care given to their loved one and to find out if information and care provided were sufficient to meet family needs [30]. A visit to the ICU after critical illness and death can be a way for the family to bring their time in the ICU to a close. After the death of a loved one, bereaved family members may still be faced with questions or issues and may leave the ICU unsatisfied or confused. According to McAdam and Erikson [35], a bereavement follow-up service could enhance family members' adaptation to life without their loved one and help ame-liorate negative physical and emotional reactions to unresolved grief [35]. Van der Link in their 2010 study investigating family bereavement found 35% of families reported a need for a bereavement follow-up service [34]. The main reason accord-ing to respondents was 'For remaining questions'. One respondent added that 'despite the severity of the situation, it is crucial to give the family members clear information, so they will suffer fewer problems afterwards' [34]. Follow-up ser-vices have the capacity to enhance family members' adaptation to life without their loved one and help ameliorate negative physical and emotional reactions to unre-solved grief [36]. Common features of these programs are an initial phone call, card or letter from a caregiver who knew the patient and the family, a family meeting for remaining questions and if necessary, referral to other agencies [34]. Fridh's Swedish study found that almost half of units surveyed (51%) reported that they often or almost always offer a follow-up visit, although in most cases, the bereaved family had to initiate the follow-up by contacting the ICU [36]. This does however also suggest that half of the families of patients who die in Swedish ICUs are sel-dom or never offered a follow-up visit/meeting. Where there is a lack of formal follow-up, some units use leaflets which include telephone numbers before the fam-ily leaves the unit after the patient's death [36]. Another important advantage of such follow-ups is that they may lead to improvement in the care of dying patients and their families. Without gaining knowledge from families' experiences, both good and bad, future EOLC cannot be improved [34, 35].

A dignified EOLC bundle can change and influence care of our patients at EOL. Synthesising the evidence into a sensible, continues bundle of EOLC practices results in a model demonstrating the incorporation of decisive turning points in transition from curative interventions to dignity at end-of-life measures.

References

1. Pattison N. A critical discourse analysis of provision of end-of-life care in key UK critical care documents. Nurs Crit Care. 2006;11(4):198–208.
2. Coombs MA, Addington-Hall J, Long-Sutehall T. Challenges in transition from intervention to end of life care in intensive care: a qualitative study. Int J Nurs Stud. 2012;49(5):519–27.
3. Truog RD, Campbell ML, Curtis JR, Haas CE, Luce JM, Rubenfeld GD, Kaufman DC. Recommendations for end-of-life care in the intensive care unit: a consensus statement by the American College of Critical Care Medicine. Cri Care Med. 2008;36(3):953–63.
4. Ramasamay Venkatasalu M, Whiting D, Cairnduff K. Life after the Liverpool Care Pathway (LCP): a qualitative study of critical care practitioners delivering end-of-life care. J Adv Nurs. 2015;71(9):2108–18.
5. Crunden E, Boyce C, Woodman H, Bray B. An evaluation of the impact of the ventilator care bundle. Nurs Crit Care. 2005;10(5):242–6.
6. Kourouche S, Buckley T, Van C, Munroe B, Curtis K. Designing strategies to implement a blunt chest injury care bundle using the behaviour change wheel: a multi-site mixed methods study. BMC Health Serv Res. 2019;19(1):1–17.
7. Capoccia G, Kelemen RD. The study of critical junctures: theory, narrative, and counterfactuals in historical institutionalism. World Polit. 2007;59(3):341–69.
8. Chavez G, Richman IB, Kaimal R, Bentley J, Yasukawa LA, Altman RB, Chen JH. Reversals and limitations on high-intensity, life-sustaining treatments. PLoS One. 2018;13(2):e0190569.
9. Back AL, Trinidad SB, Hopley EK, Edwards KA. Reframing the goals of care conversation: "we're in a different place". J Palliat Med. 2014;17(9):1019–24.
10. Curtis JR, Treece PD, Nielsen EL, Gold J, Ciechanowski PS, Shannon SE, Engelberg RA. Randomized trial of communication facilitators to reduce family distress and intensity of end-of-life care. Am J Respir Crit Care Med. 2016;193(2):154–62.
11. Curtis JR, Engelberg RA, Wenrich MD, Shannon SE, Treece PD, Rubenfeld GD. Missed opportunities during family conferences about end-of-life care in the intensive care unit. Am J Respir Crit Care Med. 2005;171(8):844–9.
12. Curtis JR, Ciechanowski PS, Downey L, Gold J, Nielsen EL, Shannon SE, Treece PD, Young JP, Engelberg RA. Development and evaluation of an interprofessional communication intervention to improve family outcomes in the ICU. Contemp Clin Trials. 2012;33(6):1245–54.
13. Wubben N, van den Boogaard M, van der Hoeven JG, Zegers M. Shared decision-making in the ICU from the perspective of physicians, nurses and patients: a qualitative interview study. BMJ Open. 2021;11(8):e050134.
14. Ahrens T, Yancey V, Kollef M. Improving family communications at the end of life: implications for length of stay in the intensive care unit and resource use. Am J Crit Care. 2003;12(4):317–24.
15. Benbenishty J, Hannink JR. Non-verbal communication to restore patient-provider trust. Intensive Care Med. 2015;41:1359–60.
16. Benbenishty J, Biswas S. Cultural competence in critical care: case studies in the ICU. J Mod Educ Rev. 2015;5(7):723–8.
17. Benbenishty J. A meaningful closure. Intensive Care Med. 2014;40:1758–9.
18. Endacott R, Boyer C, Benbenishty J, Bennun MB, Ryan H, Chamberlain W, Ganz FD. Perceptions of a good death: a qualitative study in intensive care units in England and Israel. Intensive Crit Care Nurs. 2016;36:8–16.

19. Hov R, Hedelin B, Athlin E. Good nursing care to ICU patients on the edge of life. Intensive Crit Care Nurs. 2007;23(6):331–41.
20. Barwise A, Jaramillo C, Novotny P, Wieland ML, Thongprayoon C, Gajic O, Wilson ME. Differences in code status and end-of-life decision making in patients with limited English proficiency in the intensive care unit. Mayo Clin Proc. 2018;93(9):1271–81.
21. Adams JA, Bailey DE Jr, Anderson RA, Thygeson M. Finding your way through EOL challenges in the ICU using adaptive leadership behaviours: a qualitative descriptive case study. Intensive Crit Care Nurs. 2013;29(6):329–36.
22. Holm MS, Fålun N, Gjengedal E, Norekvål TM. Music during after-death care: a focus group study. Nurs Crit Care. 2012;17(6):302–8.
23. Coombs MA. The mourning before can anticipatory grief theory inform family care in adult intensive care. Int J Palliat Nurs. 2010;16(12):580–4.
24. Coetzee SK, Klopper HC. Compassion fatigue within nursing practice: a concept analysis. Nurs Health Sci. 2010;12(2):235–43.
25. Bramley L, Matiti M. How does it really feel to be in my shoes? Patients' experiences of compassion within nursing care and their perceptions of developing compassionate nurses. J Clin Nurs. 2014;23(19–20):2790–9.
26. Martins C, Basto ML. Relieving the suffering of end-of-life patients: a grounded theory study. J Hosp Palliat Nurs. 2011;13(3):161–71.
27. Fridh I, Forsberg A, Bergbom I. Doing one's utmost: nurses' descriptions of caring for dying patients in an intensive care environment. Intensive Crit Care Nurs. 2009;25(5):233–41.
28. Benbenishty J, Bennun M, Lind R. Qualitative analysis of European and Middle East intensive care unit nursing death rituals. Nurs Crit Care. 2020;25(5):284–90.
29. Benbenishty J. Family support group: a tool for nurses. Nurs Crit Care. 2015;6(20):282–3.
30. Wessman BT, Sona C, Schallom M. Improving caregivers' perceptions regarding patient goals of care/end-of-life issues for the multidisciplinary critical care team. J Intensive Care Med. 2017;32(1):68–76.
31. Gerritsen RT, Hofhuis JG, Koopmans M, van der Woude M, Bormans L, Hovingh A, Spronk PE. Perception by family members and ICU staff of the quality of dying and death in the ICU: a prospective multicenter study in The Netherlands. Chest. 2013;143(2):357–63.
32. Kirshbaum-Moriah D, Harel C, Benbenishty J. Family members' experience of intensive care unit support group: qualitative analysis of intervention. Nurs Crit Care. 2018;23(5):256–62.
33. Efstathiou N, Walker W. Intensive care nurses' experiences of providing end-of-life care after treatment withdrawal: a qualitative study. J Clin Nurs. 2014;23(21–22):3188–96.
34. van der Klink MA, Heijboer L, Hofhuis JG, Hovingh A, Rommes JH, Westerman MJ, Spronk PE. Survey into bereavement of family members of patients who died in the intensive care unit. Intensive Crit Care Nurs. 2010;26(4):215–25.
35. McAdam JL, Erikson A. Bereavement services offered in adult intensive care units in the United States. Am J Crit Care. 2016;25(2):110–7.
36. Fridh I, Forsberg A, Bergbom I. End-of-life care in intensive care units: family routines and environmental factors. Scand J Caring Sci. 2007;21(1):25–31.

GPSR Compliance

The European Union's (EU) General Product Safety Regulation (GPSR) is a set of rules that requires consumer products to be safe and our obligations to ensure this.

If you have any concerns about our products, you can contact us on ProductSafety@springernature.com

In case Publisher is established outside the EU, the EU authorized representative is:

Springer Nature Customer Service Center GmbH
Europaplatz 3
69115 Heidelberg, Germany

The manufacturer's authorised representative in the EU is Springer
Nature Customer Service Centre GmbH, Europaplatz 3, 69115 Heidelberg,
Germany. If you have any concerns regarding our products, please
contact ProductSafety@springernature.com

Printed and bound by CPI Group (UK) Ltd, Croydon, CR0 4YY

24/04/2026

02096356-0002